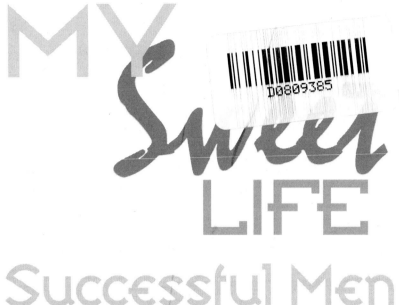

MY Sweet LIFE
Successful Men with Diabetes

Beverly S. Adler, PhD, CDE, *Editor*

Foreword by Steven V. Edelman, MD

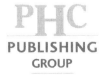

PHC
PUBLISHING
GROUP

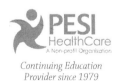

Continuing Education
Provider since 1979

PHC Publishing Group is an imprint of PESI HealthCare

2012 Eau Claire, Wisconsin

For information on this book and other continuing education
materials from **PHC Publishing Group** or **PESI HealthCare**
please call **800-843-7763**
or visit our websites
www.phcpublishing.com
www.pesihealthcare.com

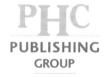

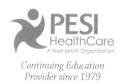

Continuing Education
Provider since 1979

PHC Publishing Group is an imprint of PESI HealthCare

Cover art by Jeff Meyer | www.ana-seer.com

A portion of the proceeds from the sale of this book will be donated, on behalf of the editor and the contributing writers, to the American Diabetes Association.

DEDICATION

This book is dedicated, in loving memory, to the three most important men who have graced my life: my father, Dr. Helmut E. Adler (1920-2001), my brother, Barry Peter Adler (1945-2009), and my beloved soul mate, Dr. Daniel Bruno (1954-2007). Each man supported my dreams, encouraged my goals, and shared in the joy of my accomplishments. They are dearly missed.

Until we meet again.

ACKNOWLEDGEMENTS

First and foremost, I want to express my deepest gratitude to my twenty-five contributing authors for sharing their life stories. While each story is unique to each author, they share the common bond of triumph over diabetes. These successful men are inspirational in their achievements yet humble about accepting any kudos as role models. They share their struggles, their strengths, their insights, and their spirituality with the reader. I also want to especially acknowledge and thank Dr. Steven V. Edelman for writing the Foreword to this book. All these men are leaders; by example, they show how to turn a "negative" diagnosis into a positive life influence.

I also would like to express my sincere thanks to my back cover endorsers, Dr. William Polonsky, Howard Steinberg, and Gary Hall, Jr., for their time and dedication to review the chapters. I appreciate their words of praise for this project.

My book would not be the collection of life stories that it is without the support of my publisher, PHC Publishing Group—Heidi Strosahl Knower has provided the most encouragement to me as I've pursued this project. Heidi and the team at PESI HealthCare recognize the positive impact that a book like this has to offer. They have my heartfelt appreciation for all their support. Special thanks to Karen Welch for her editing, and to Jillian Larson and Mike Barrickman for their support and encouragement during AADE 2012.

I would very much like to thank, my friend and colleague, Susan Weiner, RD, MS, CDE, CDN, Registered Dietician and Certified Diabetes Educator for serving as my peer reviewer. She made time in her busy schedule to read and review each chapter for clarity and correctness of content. Her comments helped to assure the highest quality of factual information.

I would also like to thank my friend and photo editor, Jeanne Dippel, for the many hours of work she completed managing the authors' photos. Her assistance was greatly appreciated.

I would like to thank my sweet suite partner, Alfred Lewis, LCSW, for his words of wit and wisdom throughout this process.

I would like to take this opportunity to acknowledge my first, most beloved, and highly esteemed diabetologist, Dr. Henry Dolger. He served for more than two decades as Chief of the Mount Sinai Diabetes Clinic and was considered a founding father of the Juvenile Diabetes Foundation. Dr. Dolger authored forty publications on diabetes, including the patient guide, *How to Live with Diabetes*, which appeared in numerous editions and languages around the world. I am honored to have these words inscribed on my copy of his book: "To Beverly. With affection, Hy Dolger." His nurturance and encouragement of my abilities to cope with diabetes were a solid source of support for me in the early years after my diagnosis.

Continued on next page...

...Continued from previous page.

I would like to thank my mother, Dr. Leonore Loeb Adler, who despite advancing age and declining health, has been supportive of my career achievements. I would also like to thank my sister and my sister-in-law for their continued moral support.

Last, but not least, I could not have accomplished what I do without the love and support of my two wonderful children, Harrison and Taylor. I am totally indebted to them for providing me with technological expertise (Harrison) and with fashion expertise (Taylor). I am as proud of them as they are of me. I am blessed to have their loving support as I pursue my professional goals.

Beverly S. Adler, PhD, CDE, *Editor*

TABLE OF CONTENTS

FOREWORD

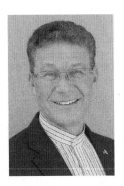

by Steven V. Edelman, MD

Celebrating the lives and stories of the struggles and triumphs of men living successfully with diabetes is so inspiring and powerful. All of the extraordinary contributing authors to this book have different lifelong experiences including the way they've turned the diagnosis of diabetes into a positive realm. Despite their individual differences, they all have one thing in common… a burning desire to succeed in life despite any challenges and to help others in any way they can. *My Sweet Life: Successful Men with Diabetes* will inspire you, and your loved ones, to embrace diabetes. The book's message, by way of example, is not to let diabetes slow you down, but rather make it a positive force in your life.

I developed diabetes when I was fifteen years old. I lost twenty pounds and experienced the classic symptoms of excessive thirst and urination. I remember being yelled at by the other kids at the drinking fountain because I took sooooooooo long. My teachers reprimanded me for falling asleep during class as I could barely keep my eyes open. As I think back on those days, it highlights the importance of educating the public about diabetes and wiping out ignorance and intolerance.

I ended up in the Intensive Care Unit and I clearly remember the nurses kept telling me repeatedly, "You could live a normal life", "You could live a normal life." I had no clue what they were talking about. However because of the way they kept saying it, I was beginning to get a little worried. I also remember attending a diabetes class that first week while in the hospital. There I was, a young naïve and ignorant teenager with newly diagnosed type 1 diabetes sitting in a room with twenty five older overweight people with type 2 diabetes. The single fact that I remember from that class in 1970 was that ketchup had a lot of sugar in it. Even at that time, my instincts told me that this was not the best learning environment for someone like me and there had to be a better way.

I eventually was discharged home on a one shot a day regimen (NPH and Regular insulins) taken in the morning and given a strict diet, using the old Exchange System, where I would weigh all of my food…what a nuisance!

I was also supposed to test my urine for glucose four times a day and keep records of everything. At first, with the help of my family and especially my mother, Joyce, I did everything by the book. But, eventually, I lost interest.

I would see my doctor every three months, have my blood and urine collected early in the morning, and then wait the usual two to three hours for the results to come back from the lab. Glucose meters and the A1c tests were not yet available. My doctor would come into the room, look at the results, and say the same thing every time, "Steve, you are doing fine. I will see you next time." Every visit to my doctor was exactly the same. I was never told what my goals of control should be and why it was so important… in a way that I understood… and as a result, my control started to slip.

It turned out that my diabetes was horribly out of control. I only wish I could have had role models like the gentlemen in this book. When I was diagnosed with diabetes, there was nobody available for me to turn to for information. It took me several years before I realized that I should do something about the fact that I probably was not doing well.

On one occasion, I decided to test my doctor because what he was saying to me at every visit just did not make sense to me. On the morning of my next appointment, I went to a donut shop and ate five donuts. I then proceeded to give my usual urine and blood samples at the office. I remember testing my own urine in the hospital bathroom and the strip turned black in about three seconds, indicating that my blood sugar was extremely high. I waited the usual two or three hours, and finally my doctor walked into the examination room holding his clipboard studying the test results. He then looked at me straight in the eye and said, "Steve… you are doing fine. I will see you next time." From that point onward, I knew I could not trust him to take care of me and I made the decision never to see him again.

The bad news was that, during those early years of poor control, I developed several complications. I immediately sought out excellent diabetes care, which prevented those complications from reaching end stage levels and allowed me to have an excellent quality of life… despite a few bumps in the road along the way.

I went to medical school at the University of California, Davis and, during my first year physiology course in 1978, I will never forget how I felt after the professor stated that "50% of all diabetics die from diabetic kidney disease within twenty years after the diagnosis." I was twenty-three years old with eight years of diabetes behind me… only twelve years left to live, I thought. My best friend, Ken Facter, always tried to comfort me by saying that at least I knew what I was going to die of.

Those early experiences motivated me to take better care of myself and to devote my career to helping people with diabetes. Ironically and tragically, Ken died suddenly of a heart attack at the age of forty. His death was a painful wake up call to me that we must live every day to the fullest and not take one second of life for granted.

After completing my medical residency, I went to the Joslin Clinic in Boston, Massachusetts for the first part of my diabetes training, where I developed lifelong friendships. I eventually ended up at the University of California in San Diego and the Veteran Affairs Medical Center and, over the past twenty-four years, I have both had the honor and privilege of serving our country's veterans living with diabetes. This is such a special population of real heroes. I gently insist that the medical residents-in-training and Endocrinology Fellows take a military history on their patients, so they can get a feeling for what these veterans went through to defend our country. Doing so, will create a bond that will help to open bi-directional communication and eventual understanding of what important barriers may be limiting their diabetes control. Getting people with diabetes (in general) to put diabetes high on their priority list is such a key component for long-term success and depends so much on individualizing our communication styles.

As a young faculty member, I spent a lot of time and energy, after the results of the DCCT (Diabetes Complication and Control Trial) were released in 1993, trying to educate healthcare professionals on how to take better care of their patients with diabetes. However, it was slow going and diabetes care was not improving fast enough at the community level. I realized that that were many barriers at that time limiting successful diabetes management. Managed care was beginning to hamper proper medical care in a major way. As a caregiver, I was fairly helpless in trying to fight the system and there was very little education directed to people with diabetes

Lastly, it took too long for information to filter down from the major research institutions to the specialists and then to the healthcare professionals, who in turn had to change their practice habits before their patients could be the recipients of a proven treatment strategy or new device or medication.

For those reasons, I started to take the most important messages directly to those who were most affected by this condition. In 1995, I had the idea of putting on a large conference for approximately one thousand people with diabetes called Taking Control of Your Diabetes (TCOYD) at the San Diego convention center focusing on education, motivation and self-advocacy. I realized early that this approach could make a significant impact on diabetes care in this country and it was a large piece of the diabetes care puzzle that was missing.

Since the beginning of TCOYD in 1995, we have been pushing these three important themes and they have never lost their importance or magnitude:

1. You have the main responsibility for taking control of your diabetes.
2. You are your own best advocate.
3. Be smart and be persistent.

Simply stating these themes is one thing but getting folks to take ownership of their health is another... and that was the challenge. At that very first conference, I realized how thirsty people with diabetes were for information about their condition and that much more was needed to be accomplished.

TCOYD became a not-for-profit organization and has steadily grown, while maintaining a high level of quality and impactful programs across the United States. Since that first conference, we have been working hard to live by our mission statement: "Guided by the belief that every person with diabetes has the right to live a healthy, happy and productive life, TCOYD educates and motivates people with diabetes to take a more active role in their condition." (For further information about TCOYD, please see my website at the conclusion of this foreword.)

As an educator, I have always felt that there needs to be a strong emphasis on motivation, along with humor, which I feel are key components to information retention and contribute to our overall success in making positive changes. Successful educational programs must have strong and clear messages about how to live a healthy life with diabetes with well-defined and attainable goals. The participants eat, laugh and listen to the speakers together and realize that diabetes crosses all socio-economic and ethnic boundaries and that they finally are in a place where they are in the majority… and not the minority.

I have also come to realize that another unmet need in diabetes care related to the "type 3" supporter (significant other of the person living with diabetes). They play such a crucial role in the ultimate success of the person with diabetes and they must be educated as well.

My goal at these conferences is to leave the attendees with hope, motivation and guidance to make realistic commitments to their health that day. At the end of the day, the participants are so motivated that they are happy they have diabetes! This last sentence may sound funny, but it has tremendous implications.

The successful men in this book are wonderful examples of that same determination and commitment to their health. The contributing authors, like me, found their own inner strength to achieve big dreams. *My Sweet Life: Successful Men with Diabetes* is an uplifting compilation of incredible adventures that will make you look at diabetes quite differently. The honesty and drive exemplified in these chapters are a testimony to the human spirit to turn the challenge of diabetes into a triumph. It should leave the reader with hope and motivation and inspiration to commit to a healthy and happy diabetes life.

www.TCOYD.org

Publisher and Editor's note: *The foreword, submitted by Steven V. Edelman, MD, is adapted from the address Dr. Edelman delivered as the recipient of the American Diabetes Association's Outstanding Educator in Diabetes Award for 2009. He delivered the address in June 2009 at the Association's 69th Annual Meeting and Scientific Sessions in New Orleans, La. Portions reprinted with permission from Diabetes Spectrum®, Vol. 23, 2010; 202-206, Copyright 2010 American Diabetes Association.*

INTRODUCTION

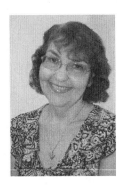

by Beverly S. Adler, PhD, CDE

My Sweet Life: Successful Men with Diabetes is filled with testosterone dripping from every page. As one contributing author says: "Testosterone is wonderful stuff." The twenty-five contributing authors to these chapters share their raw emotion as they fight their diabetes. One author describes diabetes as an "800-pound diabetes ape" that he learned to control. Another author expressed his rationale for participating in endurance events: "It gave me the opportunity to kick diabetes in the teeth with every single pedal stroke I took. It was not only addictive, but liberating—a way to shed the shackles that diabetes had attempted to place on my life. On my spirit." Yet another author wrote about his diabetes as a "ball and chain attached to my ankle that goes with me every step of my life." As a triathlon competitor, he warned his diabetes:

> It better be able to swim because I am going to drown it pulling it 2.4 miles in the ocean. And it better have thick skin because I'm going to rip every bit of its flesh off its body dragging it on the asphalt at 22 mph for 112 miles on the bike. It better have strong bones because I'm going to break every bone in its body slamming it on the ground behind me running the 26.2-mile marathon. I will use every muscle, fiber, cell, calorie, and follicle in my body to get to that finish line and collapse in the arms of the race officials. But I always have just enough strength to turn around at the finish line and step on the neck of my diabetes chained to my ankle and say "you are messing with the wrong guy!"

After my first book *My Sweet Life: Successful Women with Diabetes* was published, I was asked by many men: "Where's *our* book?" To be honest, I hadn't even thought about working on such a book. But, the outcry was so overwhelming that I had to reconsider the idea. After I did some research, I realized why this topic of men with diabetes was so necessary. There is no such collection of men's stories to be found! While women with diabetes have a website devoted to our sisterhood, there is no comparable website devoted to the brotherhood of men with diabetes. This book is the first of its type: stories of triumph for men with diabetes written by Successful Men with Diabetes. The diversity of men's stories should appeal to the diversity of men living with this chronic illness. The men who grace this book are amazing people with diabetes doing amazing things every day.

As a clinical psychologist and Certified Diabetes Educator, the therapy which I provide in my private practice focuses on the emotional adjustment of my patients to their diagnosis of diabetes. Going one step further, I've combined my career as a "diabetes psychologist" and integrated it with my personal life as a person living with type 1 diabetes (thirty-seven years). I have a unique perspective from which to free my patients from their isolation, and, at the same time, empower them. It's one thing for a therapist without diabetes to offer advice to a patient, but it's quite different when advice comes from somebody who shares that chronic illness. There is an immediate common bond which my patients appreciate. I'm somebody who "really understands how miserable a *hypoglycemic reaction* feels!" I believe that having diabetes is my blessing in disguise. I am grateful that I was diagnosed with diabetes after 1921, when life-saving insulin was first discovered. Thanks to diabetes, I live a healthy lifestyle. And last but not least, diabetes became the focus of my career. My patients and I can share diabetes stories together. While I am honest to say that I am not "perfect" with my diabetes management (nobody is!) I feel that I am a good role model to my patients.

My approach to therapy is to figuratively put my arm around my patients' shoulders rather than point a finger of blame at their diabetes management. They feel cared-for and safe without feeling guilty and judged. That is my plan for this book as well. I hope the reader will feel my arm around his shoulder and feel supported. I want the reader to feel self-confident in his self-care as well as in his personal and professional life. Diabetes is the constant thread that weaves throughout our lives. We may want to deny it, but nonetheless, diabetes is not going away. The sooner we acknowledge and accept its presence, the healthier we will be. One author expressed this sentiment of acceptance simply as, "It is what it is." Another author credited the successful management of his diabetes by actively taking action toward good health rather than responding in reaction to ill health. Diabetes, he said, taught him that he has to get up and act in order to control his life. He recognized that if he doesn't act, he will definitely have to *react* to diabetes controlling him.

Dr. Elliot Joslin (1869 - 1962) understood the key to diabetes self-care was positive action. He was the first doctor in the U.S. to specialize in the care of patients with diabetes. Dr. Joslin recognized that managing tight control of one's blood sugar through diet, exercise and insulin could extend one's life and prevent complications. He created a three-horse chariot to reflect his philosophy of living with diabetes—the three-horse motif symbolized insulin, diet and exercise, which are needed to achieve control over diabetes. I've seen educators who use three balls, juggled in the air simultaneously, to demonstrate the interaction of the three components of diabetes care.

One contributing author takes this idea of the triangular facets of diabetes self-care to a new level—a square! In his paradigm, diabetes management has four points: medication (insulin), diet, exercise, and spirituality. With all due respect to Dr. Joslin, this book supports the newer four-pronged approach to diabetes care.

As a cognitive-behavioral therapist, my therapy approach helps patients change their negative cognitions (thoughts) and behaviors (actions) to positive ones. Dr. Joslin focused on taking positive actions. I would like to discuss how your positive (or negative) thoughts influence your positive (or negative) feelings. Here's a brief lesson in the A-B-C's of cognitive-behavior therapy. "A" is the Antecedent—it is the event that occurs. It cannot be changed. In this case developing diabetes is the antecedent. "B" is the Beliefs—your thoughts, which can be unreasonable/irrational or reasonable/rational. "C" is the Consequence— how you feel emotionally, based on "B".

There is a high rate of depression among people with diabetes. Some studies suggest that diabetes doubles the risk of depression. However, newer research questions whether the symptoms of depression would be better defined as diabetes-related distress. This book is not meant as a substitute for medical care or psychiatric evaluation, but as a means to help improve your emotional well-being. If you are feeling depressed (or distressed) about "A" (the event which cannot be changed), such as dealing with daily diabetes demands, then you have to ask yourself what thoughts ("B") do you have about diabetes self-care ("A")? If they are unreasonable/irrational thoughts, you might be thinking, *"if I ignore my diabetes, then I won't be upset by it, or angry at it, or scared of it,"* etc. Ignoring diabetes (also known as denial) is not helpful to gain control over your illness. You will still have diabetes - but it will remain uncontrolled until you choose to think differently. When you change your thoughts ("B") then you can change the outcome at "C" (your feelings). A more reasonable/rational thought might be, *"I'm not happy that I have to pay attention to my diabetes, but checking my blood sugar, or counting carbohydrates, or taking a walk, etc. will help me to stay healthy."* As one of the contributing authors said "attitude will get you everywhere"! Another author declared, "Type 1 diabetes equipped me with this positive forward-looking attitude that helped turn obstacles into opportunities with even more positive outcomes."

Just who are the men in this book? They are men with incredible drive and determination to succeed in life. One author described his life with diabetes as pushing his limits—"living life at 110%, often out-distancing people with working pancreases." They are men who have learned about giving back to society. One learned "philanthropy" at a young age when he gave away the Halloween candy he collected to children who were unable to go out trick-or-treating yet were healthy enough to eat candy. Some give back in the form of involvement with kids and diabetes camps. Some give back in third-world countries where diabetes supplies and care are terribly limited. Some give online support and education in the form of blogs or podcasts. Some provide medical care or legal aid to fight diabetes discrimination. Some use their God-given talents to challenge themselves, and inspire others, with their athletic prowess. Some make a difference by using their creativity to design smart medical device innovations to make living with diabetes easier, or create healthy recipes and nutritious meals to help combat the epidemic of diabetes and obesity. These men are husbands, fathers, sons, brothers, grandpas, and uncles who also have type 1, type 1.5, or type 2 diabetes. All these men discussed how they struggled with their own diabetes management and ultimately learned not to define themselves by diabetes but rather to manage it while living their lives. As one author stated, he lives by this adage: "Diabetes—it's just a word, not a sentence!" These men are geographically located across the U.S., Canada, and across the globe. (As a side note: I kept the English spelling and terminology used by the international contributors, as we appreciate and respect everybody's differences.)

I hope the reader will enjoy these heartwarming stories filled with honesty, humor, and emotion and be inspired to "never settle for ordinary." I appreciate the authors for candidly sharing their struggles, self-doubts, and ultimate triumphs. Their stories are truly inspiring. I'm so proud to include all these men's stories in my book! I wish to all who read this book—and to all my authors who contributed to it—good health, peace, and love along your personal journey.

www.AskDrBev.com

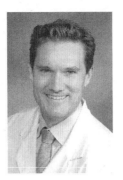

Photo credit by Weill Cornell Medical College

CHAPTER 1   *by Jason C. Baker, MD*

Surviving, and Thriving, with Diabetes

The Medical Student Who Knew Too Little

It all started with a bout of diarrhea. I was a rising third-year medical student, eager for new experiences. My sense of youthful infallibility had not yet been pierced by any substantial health crisis, and at the age of twenty-five I was physically in my prime. I was finishing a summer project in Tbilisi, Republic of Georgia, where I had worked for six weeks, researching the prevalence of HIV and hepatitis C in patients with tuberculosis. It had been my first time in the developing world, a turning point in my life that would give birth to a love of international medicine. Besides a mean battle with jet lag, I had felt excellent while working in Tbilisi. But in the last week of my rotations, I developed a fever and chills, then BAD diarrhea. I attributed it all to bad borscht that I had eaten the day before. To my chagrin, I spent my last two nights in Tbilisi confined on the couch of the pre-Soviet apartment that the medical school had arranged for me, blearily gazing up at the resplendent ornamentation of woodwork and crystal chandelier from another era, then shifting my gaze to the veranda beyond which a burned-out car lay from a more recent era. Little did I know that this fever would herald a new era for me.

I returned to Atlanta to begin my third year of medical school, starting the first of a year-long series of intense clinical rotations. During my first rotation, general surgery, I lost *a lot* of weight. But I was working hard! It was totally explainable. When I had to leave multiple times to go to the bathroom, I explained away symptoms with self-diagnosis, as all medical students do: "Psychogenic polydipsia," I concluded. It was clearly all in my head. But I was starving; I just couldn't eat enough! When I was tired after meals, I concluded that I had not been getting enough sleep and was studying too hard. And I had "six-pack abs"—a clear sign of health that I attributed to a daily regime at the gym and a fast metabolism. Looking back, I cringe at my poor diagnostic skills as a student. There is a reason for the saying, "Physician, [don't] heal thyself." But like so many of us, I was unwilling to see the obvious. Although surrounded by medicine and its promise of cures, I simply couldn't face the fear of real illness.

By the time I started my pediatric rotation, I had dwindled to a shadow of my former self. I was forty pounds thinner, a veritable skeleton. The corners of my mouth were so dry they sometimes bled when I smiled, leaving larger, dry, herpetic-looking sores. My appearance, in fact, made the children shy away from the "scary" doctor even more than normal. Some would even cry when I entered their rooms. Any interest in becoming a pediatrician was dashed; it seemed I just didn't connect with kids. During the oral examination at the end of my rotation, to the horror of my proctor, I actually nodded off. My grades suffered. Rumors circulated that I was on drugs. No one thought diabetes. No one. Least of all me.

When my mouth sores finally got bad enough, I went to a dermatologist who diagnosed me with "fungal angular chelitis." She prescribed a topical ointment that seemed to help. To her credit, the dermatologist seemed quite concerned with my general health and suggested I see a primary care doctor. Yet still no mention of "the big D."

Two months after I returned to Atlanta from Tbilisi, Grandma Baker came to town. Grandma Baker was a force to reckon with who had always been so proud that I had gone to medical school. She had wanted to be a nurse herself, but her family and circumstances in depression-era Minnesota demanded a different path. But now, escorted by my father and his partner, she had made the difficult trip to see me in action: to attend a few classes, tour the hospital, even take a spin in the cadaver lab (to which grandma has since donated her body). When I arrived to greet her at their hotel, my green scrubs hanging on the beanpole of my body, grandma immediately dragged me to the hotel breakfast bar to "fatten me up." She pumped me full of orange juice and muffins, cereal and waffles. "Jay-Jay," she exclaimed, "Honey, you've got to get some meat on those bones!" To this day, I joke about the morning grandma tried to kill me with carbohydrates.

At many medical schools, medical students in their first two years of training see each other almost daily at lectures and various meetings. Yet when they enter into clinical rotations during their third and fourth years, they might go months without seeing one another. Just after my two-month pediatric rotation finished, the class gathered together for a lecture. Faces turned toward me as I entered the lecture hall, attempting to hide surprise and concern but failing miserably in the effort. I even heard a whisper of "AIDS?" At that moment, my best friend Brooke approached, and in an attempt to diffuse the tension, announced in her tremendously bubbly tone, "Call 911! Somebody stole Jason's butt!" I was angry at the remark—hurt actually, as I thought I was looking quite cut and model-like. After the lecture, Brooke timidly approached again, this time with a friend's sincere concern. "Jason, are you all right?" Refusing to take "yes" for an answer, she continued, "You need to see a doctor." I remember being annoyed by the suggestion. I suspected the trip to the waiting room of the student health clinic would suck several hours of my time. But as luck would have it, I remembered that it was the Monday before Thanksgiving. Many of the often-sick undergraduates already would have left campus for their respective happy homes. I might be called quickly into the doctor's office and done in a matter of minutes. I could even hit the gym before the afternoon was out. I protested my health to Brooke one last time, then finally agreed to the trip. Within a few hours, my life changed forever.

Finding Control with God

666 mg/dL! That was my glucose at diagnosis. I was ushered into the emergency room where I knew the head physician. Not one to miss a teaching opportunity, the physician gave me a text to read on *diabetic ketoacidosis* even as he began treating my own with insulin and fluids. I spent two sleepless, stunned nights in the hospital, where the concepts of fingerstick tests and injection techniques were pounded (or pricked) into my consciousness. I remember being especially daunted by the notion of carbohydrate counting. I lay awake at night feeling alone and scared and extraordinarily sorry for myself. I ultimately turned to God, asking that all-too-common question: "Why me?" I soon realized I had never been alone. At that moment the words "Sink or swim, Jason," entered my mind. Tough love. And I was determined to swim.

Of course, I didn't know then that I would need various lifejackets over the next few years as I waded into the choppy waters of diabetes. In the months that followed, I was also diagnosed with aplastic anemia and told that, without a bone marrow transplant, I might die. I went into action mode, trying to busy myself with tasks to dull the fear. I fretted over everything from who would pay back my student loans (given my parents had been co-signers), to the life experiences I had never had the chance to have. I vowed that, if given the opportunity, I would live more fully. Still, I knew that magical thinking wouldn't stave off the inevitable. Two bone marrow biopsies followed, then a trip to the National Institutes of Health. I can still hear the crunching noise as the needle was drilled into my hip bone, still feel the inexplicable internal tugging sensation as the aspirate of bone marrow was taken. My toes curled. My teeth gnashed. I was informed that my body had been in a starvation state. My bone marrow had nearly been destroyed in the process. But by some grace, it had survived. My bone marrow would recover. And so would I. It had been a second brush with death, a second shock of mortality. Somehow, I had again faced death and come out on top. I felt there had to be a purpose for the diagnosis. A meaning in this second battle. A reason for my survival. A change was in order, not only in theory but also in practice.

By the time I entered my third year in medical school, plumper, healthier, and with a good deal more perspective, a sense of clarity had entered my life. I worked hard to give up control over things I could not control. I decided to use my own experience as inspiration for my studies. Diagnosis had come just at the moment when I would need to decide my field of expertise. Perhaps the illness that made pediatrics impossible might make the field of diabetes care the perfect place for me. Whether it had been there all along, or whether I had made it for myself, I ultimately found meaning in my diagnosis—by devoting myself professionally to the care of others living with diabetes.

I felt that I had not been alone in facing the challenge of diabetes, nor would I feel alone should any other medical issue arise. I continue to draw from this source of comfort with all aspects of my life, including the daily challenges of diabetes.

Losing Control with Hypoglycemia

I remember my first bad low blood sugar reaction. It hit me so fast. I was in a psychiatry lecture ten days after diagnosis and finding it extremely hard to concentrate. (That is, harder than usual.) I remember Brooke at my side, watching as I stared blankly at the instructor. I must have looked pale; I never did ask her, but I felt "funny." Still new to the process, I finally realized I needed to check my blood sugar. I was not yet comfortable doing so in public, so I stood up during the middle of the lecture, walked rather awkwardly into the corridor, then stopped. Brooke was immediately at my side. I remember her distant-sounding words that didn't make sense at the time: "Let's check your blood sugar." She helped prick my finger, then applied my blood to the strip. 22 mg/dL. "Oh my, Jay," she said. "We need some sugar." I remember turning dumbly to the vending machine next to us. "Darn," Brooke muttered as she fumbled for change, rushed it into the machine. Finally I felt a cold can in my hands, the drink on my lips, and precious sugar in my mouth. It took five minutes of relative silence for my senses to return enough for me to speak. When I looked at Brooke's stricken face, I smiled. We both broke into hysterical nervous laughter.

Of course, everyone has more than one bad experience. My next bad low blood sugar reaction happened at the dentist. I had booked the appointment by playing the "diabetes card." Realizing that I was a year overdue for my "six-month cleaning," and hoping to skip ahead of the dentist's five-month waiting list, I exclaimed, "but I have diabetes, and I'm at risk for dental and gum disease." I was seen the following day. I was on NPH and Regular insulins at the time and had given myself the routine morning shot. Halfway through the cleaning I started to feel funny, but I was embarrassed about going low ("bad diabetic!"). I ignored the early warning symptoms, determined to simply wait it out. As I lay on the chair, the dentist looming over me, his polishing brush replete with gritty paste, I felt my pulse quicken and my skin grow sweaty. Finally, fearing a low blood sugar reaction like the one I had had a few weeks earlier, I interrupted the dentist, excusing myself "to go to the bathroom." I didn't have sugar on me at the time ("bad diabetic!") so I made my way toward the vending machine I had seen in the lobby. That's where the *hypoglycemia* really hit hard. All I could envision was the Coke® that had revived me before. Through my haze, I somehow found coins in my pockets that I hastily pumped into the machine. I pushed the button, but to my horror, nothing happened. No soda. I panicked, turned toward an adjacent candy machine. I remembered the Mentos® commercial I had seen that morning before leaving home. A few coins, the button, and finally the sugar I needed. I pumped my mouth full of an entire sleeve of the minty saviors before returning to the dentist's chair. His handiwork decidedly undone, the dentist gave me a scathing look, then sighed and started over.

Through these first experiences, I realized how easy it could be for me to let my embarrassment over *hypoglycemic reactions* wrench away my control of diabetes. I also realized that I needed to make sure I had the resources to detect and treat low blood sugars on me at all times. I began to watch for early symptoms of *hypoglycemia* and treat early. I learned, over time, to share the symptoms of *hypoglycemia* with the person I was with to avoid misinterpretation of my mood and actions. I still have *hypoglycemic reactions* but, with frequent monitoring of my blood sugar, I have learned to catch my low blood sugar before it catches me.

Prick Me

Nothing, absolutely nothing, has provided me more power over my diabetes than fingersticks. I am blessed with the resources to not have to ration fingerstick supplies, so if I feel "off," I check. I check so often that frequently I know I'm "off" without even checking. I am still wrong sometimes, though, so I have learned to trust the machine over my own intuition. I often think about how beautiful a pancreas is, constantly monitoring and adjusting insulin release in concert with blood sugar fluxes. I like to think I do a pretty good job as a pancreas. I often hear comments such as "how do you check so much?" or "why do you check so much?" or simply "you check too much." Truthfully, diabetes must be personalized so that the quality of life of someone with diabetes can be at its highest. For me, that quality of life is achieved through peace of mind with knowledge, not guess work. Knowing that my blood sugar is within my target range helps me to know that I am in control, and it has been key to helping me prevent health complications related to diabetes.

Choking on Bulimia

Prior to "the big D," I had considered myself to be in good shape, and in general felt as though I had control over my life. Diabetes, initially, changed that. I was so conscious of carbohydrate counting in the beginning, to the point of inducing intense guilt over my failure if I had "mismatched" my insulin/carbohydrate ratio. I found myself angry and anxious, constantly worrying that all of my high blood sugars were wreaking havoc on my blood vessels, nerves, and cells, and perhaps leading to damage, blindness, neuropathy, kidney failure.

I never actually had a sweet tooth prior to my diabetes diagnosis, passing up the most delectable-looking desserts without so much as a blink. The limitations of diabetes made me "want what I couldn't have." I began to experiment with desserts, especially ice cream. The problem was that I found myself enjoying those sweet treats too much and soon lost control of the concept of portions. I would buy a half-gallon of sugar-free ice cream (which is certainly not carbohydrate free) and found myself eating the entire thing in one sitting. Racked with guilt after, and knowing that my blood sugar was rising, but not wanting to give more insulin out of fear of weight gain, I discovered I could force myself rather efficiently to throw up what I had eaten. What a neat trick; I could indeed have it all! Soon I was doing this, not only with desserts but with all foods. I found myself gravitating toward buffets, where I indulged in all types of foods that I knew would spike my blood sugar based on the portions I ate. Bulimia was a fix, and it gave me a sense of control over my diabetes—a false sense of empowerment that continued for two years after my diagnosis.

Intellectually, I knew this was not good practice. I knew that the action was hard on my throat, my teeth, and ultimately my psyche as the cycle of guilt and pleasure began to isolate me. Finally I shared my secret with Nancy, a dear friend from my internal medicine residency class at New York University. Nancy and I enjoyed a love of good food and, to the chagrin of our thin wallets, often savored many of the culinary delights offered in New York. Nancy looked at me calmly, not judging, and as I said the words to her, I cried, feeling a release of the isolation and guilt that had built up over the prior two years. Nancy said to tell her of the urges as they arose so she could help me to diffuse them. It took two more years of struggle to get my bulimia under control. Through this experience, I realized that I could not conquer diabetes alone; I needed to draw upon the love and guidance of friends and family. I realized that, until I was open about my struggles with diabetes, it would control me rather than I it.

Doctor or Patient?

Medical training can be grueling, in particular the clinical rotations, which often deprive one of sleep, exercise, and ready access to healthy foods. All too often, doctors in training going through this process lose sight and control of their own lives and health as they try to guide and heal the lives of others. Diabetes grounded me in the process. Soon after my diagnosis, I knew that my health had to be a priority and that I couldn't care for anyone else unless I cared for myself. This was a good theory that reality didn't always allow me to practice, however. Emergency situations warranted immediate action, which often didn't translate into good diabetes control. Case in point: I had *just taken* my injection for an already hurried meal when the announcement of "code red" (crashing patient) echoed overhead. I had to rush to the critically ill patient's bedside, so I "wolfed down" my meal, overcompensating for a potential *hypoglycemic reaction*, given the unknown of how long it would be before I could next check my blood sugar (this was in the era before reliable continuous glucose monitors). I knew I would be useless if I crashed next to the crashing patient. The adrenaline, paired with the over-compensated glycemic load, proved very challenging toward controlling my glucose levels. I found my blood sugar frequently swinging both high and low.

I became angry and frustrated with diabetes and resentful toward a medical career that forced me to sacrifice my own health in order to help that of others. I never thought I would drop out of the medical world, but I began to doubt any designs I had on becoming an endocrinologist. How could I live AND work constantly amidst the subject of diabetes? I would lose my mind! I began, again, to let diabetes control my life. As I began to share my frustrations and doubts with others in my residency class, I was surprised to feel a sense of clarity again present itself. Now, as an endocrinologist, I celebrate my diabetes and how it helps me connect to my patients, allowing me to help them take control of their own diabetes through my example. Indeed, each person must find his or her own path to do this, but I like to think that sharing some of my own trials and tribulations with diabetes might help others in this process.

Barely Surviving: Diabetes in the Developing World

I am blessed to have access to a wealth of resources to help control my diabetes. Sadly, this is not a universal right. My first experience with managing type 1 diabetes in the developing world was during a summer rotation I did in Ghana during my fourth year of medical school. Soon after my arrival in Ghana, I vividly remember sitting in the middle of an extremely crowded bus, choked with five people across, as it careened down a bumpy road somewhere between Accra and Kumasi. I had been doing a pretty good job of managing my diabetes prior to arriving in Ghana, and I had a nice and stable routine going in Atlanta. I thought I had come to Ghana prepared, armed as I was with extra insulin, syringes, and test strips, along with a pile of Atkins snack bars (low carbohydrate protein bars). Sitting on the ripped dusty seat of the converted yellow school bus, I pulled out my kit and checked my blood sugar: 260 mg/dL. I had suspected it would be high, feeling a bit foggy and remembering the questionable carbohydrate content of fish sauce I had eaten earlier (despite being told it was devoid of carbohydrates by a local doctor). I was using syringes, so I drew up a few units just as the bus hit a bump on the edge of the road, swerving to avoid an overturned lumber truck (a common cause of accidents and death on the Ghanaian roadway). My fellow passengers and I were collectively catapulted a foot, as a unit, at a 45-degree angle in the air. Luckily, I had sandwiched my kit between my knees, so it didn't spill its contents onto the dusty corrugated floor, but the needle I had poised to inject savagely stabbed my abdomen. A woman seated next to me, ensconced in the typical bright Ghanaian dress replete with an elaborate head cover, gasped! I looked at her like a wounded white animal.

At least I had the insulin to inject. They had no fingerstick supplies. No A1c testing. Uncertain and erratic food supply, if available, likely comprised of starchy and glycemically unfriendly foods. If people with diabetes were lucky enough to get insulin, likely it was NPH. Welcome to type 1 diabetes in the developing world. While traveling in the developing world, each time I met another person with type 1 diabetes, I counted my blessings for the suitcase full of personal medical supplies that I enjoyed. My designer insulins, my unending glucose testing supplies. The stories I had heard and the complications I had seen motivated me to use those resources, and reminded me that there was no excuse, no barrier, against my taking charge of my diabetes. Those stories also motivated me to share my medical wealth with others not as fortunate.

One of the more poignant stories about the plight of people with type 1 diabetes was that of Marjorie, whom I met while working in Uganda in 2010. Marjorie was three years old when she was diagnosed with type 1 diabetes, and just twenty-nine years old when she died, having succumbed to diabetes-related kidney failure. Unlike so many people with type 1 diabetes in Uganda and other parts of the developing world, Marjorie was one of the lucky ones. Marjorie had been provided enough insulin and glucose testing supplies to allow her to survive. Yet Uganda is starved for resources that would have allowed Marjorie to keep her blood sugar levels under good enough control to avoid diabetes complications.

While she awaited a kidney transplant—a treatment that she never received—Marjorie relied on weekly dialysis treatments to stay alive. More often than not, Marjorie could not afford such treatments and faced a preventable slow and painful death. Yet throughout this painful time, Marjorie continued her efforts to educate both patients and healthcare providers on how to better manage type 1 diabetes, in hopes of preventing others from suffering her fate.

Speaking at various medical conferences, Marjorie recounted her story and fought to change a system that had limited her own care because of a lack of resources.

Through this was born "Marjorie's Fund," a not-for-profit type 1 global diabetes initiative that I started in 2011, which aims to improve the resources and education for type 1 diabetes patients in the developing world, and to promote research toward ultimately curing and preventing this disease. The management of type 1 diabetes in the developing world can and must be improved. Without better resources, more patients like Marjorie will survive into adulthood, only to suffer and inevitably die from the many complications associated with late diagnosis and poor diabetes control. Marjorie ultimately succumbed to her complications, but with the help of Marjorie's Fund, others need not. Marjorie's Fund aims to help people living with type 1 diabetes in the developing world not only to survive diagnosis but to thrive after diagnosis, living long and healthy lives despite having diabetes. As a person with type 1 diabetes who lives in a resource-rich bubble, I have learned through the stories of others less financially fortunate that it is my obligation to use the resources I have to manage my own diabetes and to work toward helping others do the same. (For further information about Marjorie's Fund, please see the website at the conclusion of this chapter.)

Diabetes Can be a Blessing

The process of accepting my diabetes, and celebrating it, is ongoing. I often think that if I were given the option of reversing time and somehow avoiding diabetes, I would not take it. In many ways diabetes has enriched my life, enhanced my appreciation for the simple pleasures—my physical health, my spiritual health—and has given me a framework for a successful career in medicine. Diabetes can truly be a blessing. My greatest advice to any person with type 1 diabetes is to seek strength in this challenge and embrace diabetes by sharing your story and increasing awareness in others. Use the resources you are given, remembering there are many others who are far less fortunate. In so doing, you will control your diabetes rather than let it control you: not only surviving with diabetes, but thriving with diabetes!

www.marjoriesfund.org

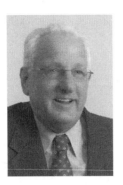

CHAPTER 2   *by Marc H. Blatstein, C.H.C., AADP*

Winning with Diabetes

My Diagnosis

I'll never forget September 1, 1960. It was a bright and sunny day—just the kind of day a ten-year-old boy would love to play outside. There was one problem that preceded that day, however; for the last three and a half months, I had been too tired to go outside much and do anything at all.

Not only was I tired but irritable, thirsty, and constantly running to the bathroom. I had been to the doctor a week before for a blood test to determine what was wrong. I was a happy-go-lucky kid who didn't worry too much about anything. My father came home early from work that day, which I thought was unusual. My mother and father asked me to sit down at the kitchen table because they had to talk to me. They proceeded to tell me I had Juvenile Diabetes. They both started to cry, and I just couldn't understand why they were so upset. The guilt I felt from their crying stayed with me for many years. I felt very bad that I upset my parents so terribly with that diagnosis.

I was sent to Children's Hospital of Philadelphia and stayed there for weeks. To this day I still don't understand why I was there so long. Dr. Robert Kay was my endocrinologist; he was also the co-founder of what eventually became the Juvenile Diabetes Research Foundation. He was a great guy and very funny, but when he told my parents that I should stay away from cake, candy, and ice cream, I thought my life was over! I told Dr. Kay that I didn't want to wear pajamas while in the hospital because they made me feel sick even though I didn't feel sick. I had a habit of making everything a big joke, and Dr. Kay asked me every morning to accompany him and the other doctors on Grand Rounds at the hospital because I made them laugh. He also brought me along because I made all of the other "sick kids" on the floor laugh. Being in the hospital was a lot of fun, I thought, although my family didn't agree.

When my parents brought me home, my mother went on a mission to find me sugar-free cake, candy, and ice cream. Remember that was back in 1960! The first day I was home my mother went out to find a "diabetic pound cake." She came home with this amazing loaf of cake, and I was ecstatic! She cut a piece and put it on a plate. I couldn't wait to take my first mouthful. As soon I put it in my mouth and swallowed it, panic set in. It was like trying to swallow a handful of sand. I said, "Mom, I thought you loved me; you're trying to kill me!" The guilt on her face was so sad. Well, no more cake for me! Her next mission took her to downtown Philadelphia to get me a box of "diabetic chocolates." My grandmother was taking care of me until she got back. When she came through the door, I almost tackled her from excitement! She opened the box of chocolates and put two perfectly shaped pieces on a plate in front of me. I picked one up and smelled it. It smelled like real chocolate. WOW!! Was I excited! I put one in my mouth and bit down. Panic set in again. This putrid, horrid sour taste almost made me vomit. The aftertaste lasted a month, I swear. My poor mom.

I found a way to get my cake, candy, and ice cream, though. I came up with a scheme to get my way with sweets. On a Saturday morning, I walked into my mother's room and told her that my blood sugar was low. She said, "I'll get you juice." I said, "No juice! Candy would work better, I just know it." Little did she know that I had been in the bathroom prior to that, smacking my cheeks and dripping water on my face. Boy, did I look like I was having a serious low blood sugar reaction. Ha!! That plan worked for not quite a month until she caught me in the bathroom prepping for my next "low." I was busted!

In the early years with diabetes, I was told a lot of what I couldn't do because I had diabetes. I, Marc H. Blatstein, was going to do whatever I could to be like a "normal" kid. In elementary school I was made fun of by a couple of kids who called me "needle feet." It upset me. I got into a number of fist fights because of it, but eventually things improved and we became friends. They improved because I kicked their butts!

"Can Do" Attitude

Getting back to Dr. Kay; he was one of my biggest cheerleaders. He always told me that I could do whatever I wanted even though I had diabetes. He instilled the "Can Do" attitude in me. I was a happy and rambunctious kid who eventually grew up to be a happy and rambunctious adult. Thank you, Dr. Kay.

As I came into my teenage years, I wanted to play more and more sports such as baseball, basketball, track, and football. When I went out for the track team in high school, my coach and parents were a little leery. The typical question everyone asked was what I would do if I had a low blood sugar reaction. So we all agreed that there would be a sugared drink close by. (Doing urine testing at the time was of no help.)

At one of the track meets, which included hurdles, I ran into a problem. I didn't drink the sugared drink as I was supposed to. I started the run and went over one hurdle, then another, then another, and that's all I remember. I woke up on the exam table in the nurse's office with her picking stones out of my knees and legs. Apparently, my blood sugar dropped so low that I didn't make it over the last hurdle. They said I passed out in mid-air. But I thought to myself, *"I still can do it!"* Before my basketball games or track meets, I recited to myself over and over, *"I can do it, I can do it!"* I was my own cheering section. At a couple of my basketball matches, I also passed out. Not deterred, I thought to myself again, *"I will continue to find a way to do it. I know I can!"* The coaches and other players went from being afraid of what might happen to me to cheering me on after I scored or won a meet. I needed to prove to myself that I was just like the other kids, but with a few of the inconviences that the other team members didn't have. My mother always called Dr. Kay to ask him if it was okay for me to play each sport. He said that I was a regular kid with a couple of extra steps that I needed to take to stay healthy. He told my mother to let me play. Thanks again, Dr. Kay.

My "Can Do" attitude started to waiver when I was around seventeen years old. It came to a head in the summer of 1969 when my best friend, Barry, and I enrolled in summer courses at a college in New Mexico.

Facing the Fear

During my teen years, my endocrinologist suggested that I see a psychologist to help me work out some of the angst and anger I was starting to feel about living with diabetes. His name was Dr. Barney Dlin. In my eyes, he was a saint. He listened, counseled, motivated, and supported me to achieve whatever I wanted to do. Thank you, Dr. Dlin.

Barry and I left for New Mexico in June of 1969. I was nineteen years old and Barry was eighteen years old. We thought we were invincible and could conquer and do anything! We signed up for the regular classes but added one to the list. It was called "Man and His Elements." This was an eight-week endurance and strength training course. Morning runs for over five miles, strength training, rope training, etc. Maybe I can't do this? Our coach/instructor/"dictator" was an ex-Marine sergeant. Does that tell you something? Every time I told him I couldn't do it because of my diabetes, he would literally kick me in the butt and tell me that he wasn't going to let my diabetes stop me from achieving anything. He said that maybe I wouldn't be a Marine, but he was going to help me achieve the Marine toughness and attitude. I give thanks to my Marine coach today. Thanks, Coach! Our final exam for this course was not a typical one. We were told that, for our final we would go up to the foothills of New Mexico, Sitting Bull Falls, to do survival training: a rock climb down a 500-foot cliff, a friction climb down the 500-foot face of another side of the cliff, and finally we would rappel with ropes down the 700-foot face of the other side. *"What did I get myself into?"* There would be no normal food—just rations—and absolute fear and pain.

The sergeant also told us to be on the watch for snakes, bears, and tarantulas. *"I'm going to die,"* I thought. I can, but maybe I can't do this? During that crazy weekend, whenever I would slow down or want to stop during our hikes, I would say that I was having a low blood sugar reaction. The sergeant would give me a candy bar, physically pick me up if I was sitting, and say: "Let's go, Blatstein! You're not quitting. There's no turning back now." The climbs were very tough, but the rappelling was blood curdling, especially since I'm afraid of heights. I got help putting on my body gear before the rappel, and I was the last one to go down the cliff face. I stood at the edge, looked down, and threw my rope over. The sergeant said: "Marc, life is all about hurdles, challenges, roadblocks and fears. Facing the fear that's stopping you now will train you to face the challenges your diabetes and life can throw at you later. The only thing you have to fear is fear itself." He then inched me back off of the cliff. As I clumsily rappelled down, I was both scared and excited. Half way down I started shouting, "I can do it! Diabetes will never stop me again!" Through the years, I've faced many challenges from life and especially from my diabetes. But that weekend prepared and showed me that I could handle anything!

My three coaches in my life with diabetes—Dr. Robert Kay, Dr. Barney Dlin and the Marine sergeant (whose name I unfortunately do not remember)— taught me to laugh through the obstacles of diabetes and life. They also taught me that I'm a fully functioning person, that there are no failures—just learning experiences—and, last but not least, that I can do anything I set my mind to do! But I don't want to leave out my biggest fan, coach, and mentor: my mother, Blanche. Without her, I might not be here today. I miss you and love you with all of my heart, Mom. THANKS!

Making a Difference

There were many people with diabetes in my family. Two who had a large impact on my life were my first cousin, Marcy, and my Aunt Ruth. Marcy lived with type 1 diabetes until the age of 77. She had diabetes for 72 years! Marcy and I were like a brother and sister. We were each other's teachers and coaches when it came to our diabetes. She passed away in 2009, and I will always miss her. My Aunt Ruth was diagnosed with type 2 diabetes around or before 1970 and unfortunately ignored it every step of the way. She passed away in 1979 when I was twenty-nine years old. She was a mother to my five cousins, a wife, a caterer, and an overall amazingly nice person. She would always have something for me to eat that was sugar-free when I came over. I loved her!

Her health went downhill, due to diabetes complications, over a ten-year period until she entered a nursing home in the late 1970s. I would visit this once vibrant woman, now in a nursing home, and it would break my heart. The last time I saw her was about a week before she passed away in October of 1979. She had lost her sight and had a multitude of other diabetes-related complications. We held hands and spoke a little. Before I was ready to leave, she said, "Marc, don't do to yourself what I did to myself, and make a difference." Later on I realized that my Aunt Ruth saved my life. Because of her, I also realized that I couldn't divorce my diabetes or fire it, so I made it my partner in life. Thank you, Aunt Ruth! I will always miss you and be thankful to you.

Because of what my Aunt Ruth said to me, I realized that I could help not only myself with my diabetes but also others. Whenever there was a diabetes support meeting or event, I would go. There I would meet others with diabetes, and we would share our stories. I also had this uncanny ability to take the most negative person with diabetes and make him or her smile and laugh.

A Major Bump in the Road

On April 29, 1984, I hit a major bump in the road with my life. It was a sunny Sunday morning, and I was setting out to help my cousin Alan move a 2000-pound wood lathe from one part of an old warehouse to another. We were on the second floor of a very high-ceilinged room. He and I each were over six feet tall, weighed near 250 pounds, and had 50 inch chests and 19 inch arms. We were thirty-four years old and felt invincible!

After moving the lathe, I walked toward the bathroom, tripped over something, and fell backwards. I thought that wouldn't be a problem because I had been a student of both Judo and Tae Kwon Do, so I knew how to fall. But it was a problem! I was falling through an open trap door to the ground over twenty feet below. I tried stopping my fall with my right arm, but I felt it pull out of the socket. I hit the concrete and lay there awake but dazed. Luckily I had put my head to my chest as I was falling so I didn't break my neck. Thoughts were racing through my head: *"How bad am I? Am I going to live? Would I ever walk again?"* There was absolutely no feeling in my body. I had to live! I had children, my wife, my family, and many friends. I absolutely refused to give up!

As I lay there, an amazing thing happened to me. There were thoughts and voices in my head that I knew didn't belong to me. In my stupor, I remember sensing at one point that I was looking down at my body. Also, the voice in my head was asking if I was ready to go home. To this day I can still feel these senses, and I still wonder what I was really experiencing. Later I thought, *"Did I really have an out-of-body experience?"*

15

The paramedics came and scraped me off the ground. I heard one of them say that he didn't think I would make it. I couldn't speak, but I was not going to quit. After a few minutes in the ambulance, the pain in my body and back became excruciating! Once at the hospital, I was rushed into the emergency room and a surgical suite. They cut off my clothes, and I heard the whispers of how bad off I was. I whispered to the doctor, "Please, pain killers!"

I woke up after surgery the next day. I was in pain all over, even though I was on pain killers. I had machines doing everything for me, including forcing me to breathe. But I had too much to live for; I had to make it!

That week is a partial blur of machines and tubes doing the work my body should have done. A few days after the accident, I awoke to find about twenty people in my room. There was supposed to be only three people at a time. I found out later that the critical care nurse and doctor had called my family and told them they didn't think I'd make it more than a few more days. I saw everyone's faces, some crying, most frowning. I patted the nurse on the shoulder to give me a writing tablet, and I wrote a note on this tablet with the only part of my body that worked—my left arm. The note said, "I've just begun to fight, don't worry!" I wanted to take their pain away. I was going to heal!

All I could do was lie there and think, day in and day out. I kept going over the accident step by step. What did I learn from all of this? What had I learned so far from having diabetes for twenty-four years?

Late in the second week, they transferred me to Jefferson Hospital Rehabilitation Center in downtown Philadelphia. The next week of my ordeal, things became even more challenging. I was put in a body cast. They laid me on a table, strapped me in, made sure my intravenous drip filled with Valium was operating, and proceeded to wrap me like a mummy. After wrapping me in this horrendous body cast, the doctors told me that I might not get back all of my mobility after I healed. Oh yes I would!

Into the third week of my hospital stay, I pestered the doctors to take me to the rehabilitation room. They said it would be a while before I could go there. I said, "I want to do it now!" I drove the staff crazy until they came in to my room one day and told me I was crazy. They said my back was broken in three places, all of my ribs were cracked, I had many contusions and abrasions, and my insides needed to heal from the abdominal surgery I had. I said, "I want to go to rehab now!" I was taken to the rehab room a few days later. Throughout the ride in the wheelchair, I must have passed out a couple of times from lightheadedness. I had had no food for almost two weeks. The only nutrition I got was through a tube in my arm. As I arrived at this enormous room, I saw many paraplegics and quadriplegics, and I said, "That won't be me!"

As they wheeled my chair in front of the rehab bars, I began to sweat. The bars looked as if they were a mile long. Can I do this? Yes I can! They again tried to convince me to stay in the chair. Again I said, "No way!" I remember pushing myself up from the chair, swaying and sweating, ready to pass out but fighting through it. The rehab doctor told me I didn't have to do this. I ignored him. I grabbed the bars and tried to walk. My legs wouldn't go. My body was wracked with pain, but in my head I said, *"I can do this!"* I dragged myself a few feet using the bars. My legs wouldn't go. I started to yell at my legs as if they were a separate being. In a few more feet of struggle, my legs started to go inch by inch. I laboriously went to the end of the bars, turned around, and made it halfway back before I passed out. I awoke on the floor to cheers and tears from the staff and others. I was told that what I had done was not possible. I didn't have the wind to answer, but inside I smiled and thanked God!

Thank You Diabetes

A few days later, an endocrinologist came into my room while my parents were there. He proceeded to tell them that "Marc's diabetes saved his life." I asked him what he meant. He said that diabetes had made me a stronger person, one who had taken this new-found strength and continued to heal from this catastrophic accident. He told me that what I had done was truly a miracle. I believe that out of something bad, the diagnosis of diabetes, came something good. I had survived and would function as a whole person again. Thank you, diabetes!

I was in both hospitals for six weeks and three days. They originally told me I would be there for approximately four months. I showed them. Upon my release, I walked out of the hospital on my own power in a body cast. I went home with three therapists of all kinds attending to my needs. After a few days, I thanked them all and sent them home. I rehabbed myself.

The First Diabetes Conference in the Middle East

There is a saying: "What you put out in the world will come back to you." I believe in that idea of *Karma*—if you do good things, good things will happen to you. In the fall of 1995, I was asked to be at a luncheon with a physician from Israel. Of course I agreed. I met an amazing endocrinologist over lunch, Dr. Pnina Vardi. She was the lead endocrinologist at the Schneider's Children Medical Center in Tel Aviv, Israel. During lunch she asked me to come to Israel the following March to be one of the co-chairs of the first diabetes conference in the Middle East. I was floored!! She didn't just ask me; she told me I couldn't say no! She had read about my work and had heard one of my taped speeches, and she insisted I accept. I looked her in the eye and knew it was a losing battle. I agreed, but after she told me she would pay any expenses, I told her I would not take money from any non-profit organization—including the hospital. She reluctantly agreed.

I asked my father, Harry, to go with me because he had type 2 diabetes. He gladly said yes. In March, we left for Israel. A welcoming committee from the hospital greeted us at the airport, and we were flattered by the pomp and circumstance. During our stay, I was asked to work with many children with diabetes, and I helped them smile and laugh with their disease the way I did. I also was interviewed on a national talk radio program and interviewed for their national magazine. I couldn't believe the whirlwind of events I was involved in, and at times it was overwhelming. My father had a perpetual smile on his face as everything unfolded.

My father and I were given a tour of the hospital and its facilities. I saw rooms where parents stayed with their child until he/she was better. In one such room, I was introduced to a family from the desert of Iraq, Bedouwin Arabs. Their son had just been diagnosed with type 1 diabetes, and an interpreter told them about my diabetes work. After a few minutes of conversation, the father got up and gave me a hug. He brought tears to my eyes when he thanked me and told me I was a gift from God. What an amazing experience.

On the day of the speech, I was exceptionally nervous, whereas back in the States, a speech like this was almost old hat. Dr. Vardi took me onto the stage, and when I looked out over this expansive multicultural audience, I was overcome with awe. I forgot to mention that Schneider Children's Medical Center was non-denominational; they treated children from any Middle Eastern country. Dr. Vardi told me that their mission was to heal and change a child's life with their cutting-edge care, no matter where they came from. I loved that! Over one thousand people were in the audience. There were physicians from Egypt, Syria, Qatar, India, Iran, Iraq, of course Israel, and too many more to mention. Many people who had children with diabetes were also in attendance.

Before I started to speak, Dr. Vardi said, "Marc, I know you're nervous. Just be who you are. You're a great speaker with a great heart and mission." I gave my speech to the most amazing audience I was ever privileged to speak to. At the end of the speech, I took a chance to share with the audience how I viewed religion and spirituality. When I finished my main speech I said to the audience,

> I would like to share with you my viewpoints on religion and spirituality. Religion is like a picture tube; someone may like channel 56, someone else channel 100, and I like channel 10. They all go to the same tube. If we are all so different, why don't I have five eyes, someone else have six legs, and yet someone else have seven ears? We're all the same. We come into this world the same way, and we leave this world the same way. Be good to each other because we're all we have!

My heart was thumping in my chest when I finished. I knew everyone there understood me because their second language was English. I looked out over the audience and saw my father beaming with pride. But there was dead silence. I thought, *"What did I do?"* As I walked off of the stage, I received a standing ovation. I was swarmed by dozens of MDs, hugging me and telling me that what I said was so true. I was invited to many of their countries, but I knew I couldn't attend because of my time commitments back home. That was the most amazing experience I ever had. I was on cloud nine. Many national Israeli politicians called me while I was in Israel and told me what a great job I had done and how I had transformed so many lives for the better. I will never, never forget that experience, and the best part was that I got to share it with my father, who is now no longer with us.

Juvenile Diabetes Research Foundation

Let's move ahead to 1997. I was forty-seven years young, a partner and co-founder in a national diabetes mail order pharmacy, and involved in a couple of other diabetes concerns. I was also appearing on many radio and television shows, and presenting on stage more times that I can remember. I sat on ten boards, nine of which were diabetes-related. But the most exciting part of this were the meetings I ran in seven area hospitals, teaching and encouraging people that they could "Win with their Diabetes." It was an amazing experience. I was then a Vice President of the Philadelphia chapter of the Juvenile Diabetes Research Foundation (JDRF). The meetings were becoming more frequent and filled with larger crowds. This was a remarkable opportunity to bring more members into this great foundation. Through these meetings, and with a great team around me, we created the largest national family walk that the JDRF had ever had.

At that time, I was also a pioneer of insulin pump technology, traveling all over the country to help thousands of people improve their lives with insulin pumps. The pump helped me gain better control of my blood sugar and achieve freedom from multiple injections. What a great experience to help so many others! My Aunt Ruth had asked me years before to make a difference, and I was certainly doing that.

A New Challenge

I needed another challenge, so I signed up at a Tae Kwon Do school. I had done Tae Kwon Do and Judo when I was a teenager and into my early 20s, so I thought, *"Why not? I can do it again."* My wife, kids, and friends all thought I was crazy. They were probably right, but this was another mountain I knew I could climb.

The first year of classes was tough because my once broken-up body was slower in responding to the many moves, jumps, punches, kicks, etc.

Daily, I would run up and down hills in the neighborhood. I persevered, and things consistently got better and better. I broke a few toes and pulled some muscles, all from training hard. Also, within those twelve months, I lost my mother, father-in-law, and my brother's father-in-law—all very kind and sweet people. Even though I was emotionally drained and detoured at times, I kept plugging along. The difference between a goal and a dream is a timetable, and I had a timetable. In my second year of Tae Kwon Do, I asked Fran Ott, my *SaBumNim* (the Korean term for "master") and my friend and teacher, if I could compete in a major tournament sometime soon. He told me to be patient because I wasn't quite ready yet.

In November of 2000, I was ready, willing, and able. Our team left for an international tournament in Mar Del Plata, a beach town in Argentina. We arrived at our destination after a complete day of traveling. After a couple of prep days of working out as a group, sightseeing, and enjoying the food and ambiance of the town, I was ready.

It was Saturday morning, November 15, 2000. I was nervous and excited and had some self doubts, but I knew that my diabetes had made me stronger, more resilient, sensitive, and full of the "Can Do" attitude. I had accepted diabetes as my life's partner a long time ago, and this partner was going to help give me the strength to succeed! At 9 a.m., all of us entered the stadium. I prepared my insulin dosage accordingly for the day.

We proceeded to do our patterns or forms. I was going to compete in the forms with a whole group of guys, different ages from different parts of the world. It was exciting but scary! We went through a process of elimination for about an hour. Three of us were left at the end of the forms part, and I took 3rd place. I DID IT!

The next part of the competition was sparring. I thought my heart was going to come out of my chest. My blood sugars were unstable. When I thought it was time for me to be called up, I drank my bottle of Coca-Cola® and waited. The only problem was that a five-minute wait turned into hours. So my blood sugar went up, I treated with insulin, and it went down. This went on for about four hours. They would ask me if I was ready, and then I'd wait some more. My *SaBumNim* finally asked me if I was ready; I was scared and excited—but ready to go. I checked my blood sugar; it was about 150 mg/dL. I drank a little bit of Coke® and prayed that I would survive this ordeal. I knew I could do it!

Adrenalin and stress are real killers. At 4 o'clock, the referee called my teacher and me to the judging tables. They told us that the only people close to my age to spar were between thirty-five and forty years of age. I looked at Mr. Ott and said, "Bring it on!"

I entered the sparring area along with a guy who was quite a bit less than forty years old. He was an Argentine, I was told, and he looked tough—as if he ate nails for breakfast. We squared off, the bell rang, and we went at it. I found out quickly that I was scoring as many points on him as he was on me. What wasn't good was that his stamina was superior to mine. Take away the fact that he was over ten years younger than I, and subtract the effects of a lifetime with diabetes, and you had my opponent. The rounds were ninety seconds long, but to me it seemed like an eternity. It became a test, not of who would score the most points, but if I would be standing at the end of each round. And I was! I stood my ground against my opponent.

We had one more round to go. I was struggling with blood sugars under 90 mg/dL. I kept drinking my Coke®, hoping that my blood sugar would come up. Mr. Ott told me that my opponent and I were tied. I was just glad I had survived so far. Mr. Ott asked if I was ready. I checked my blood sugar again and, to my dismay, it was *below* 80 mg/dL. More Coke®. I can do it! Fran told me, "You have it, Marc. Third place will be yours. Just hold on for another minute."

Could I do it? Would a fifty-year-old body hang together for one more round? Or would I fall on my face before the minute had passed? The floors were hardwood gym floors. If only I had more time for my blood sugar to recover. But I didn't, and good sense prevailed, so after a moment's thought I made a hard decision: I would walk away from third place. Better to pass up the match than to pass out during the match. "Mr. Ott," I finally said, "There's always another day, another tournament. I've already won this one. I did it. I really did it!"

This was a personal victory that I knew I had won on all counts. I had climbed another mountain in my life and had beaten back diabetes yet again. My friend and teacher, Mr. Fran Ott, always believed in me, encouraged me, and helped me climb this mountain. I want to thank him and my Tae Kwon Do family who helped me achieve this life's milestone at fifty years of age. I could not have done it without you all. Thank you.

My New Career

Let's move to the present. It's May 2012. All of the years spent doing both for-profit and non-profit work and teaching people to lead better lives with diabetes have led me to an amazing career. I've just finished my course in becoming a Certified Health Coach (C.H.C.). This schooling was provided by The Institute for Integrative Nutrition, in New York City, an organization that has graduated over 13,000 people since its inception. Its experts, who are at the forefront of wellness, are such well known people as Dr. Andrew Weil, Dr. Deepak Chopra, and many more amazing people.

After my graduation, I now have two titles: C.H.C. and AADP (member in good standing of The American Association Of Drugless Practitioners).

I now have the pleasure of working with many people with diabetes, their family members and friends whom I teach how to smile and laugh and "Win with their Diabetes" as I have. I continue to speak to and teach groups and individuals. I have many opportunities and projects within the realm of my new career. Where else can I do what I love to do so much?

50 Years with Diabetes

When I was diagnosed with type 1 diabetes, I didn't know that someday I would receive an award for living with diabetes for fifty years. The renowned Joslin Diabetes Center awarded me its 50-Year Medal. Since 1970, the Joslin Diabetes Center has presented more than three thousand 50-Year Medals across the country and around the world. I've also received the Lilly Diabetes Journey Award™, provided by Eli Lilly and Company, which recognizes diabetes patients in the U.S. who have successfully managed their disease for fifty years with the help of insulin.

Type 1 Diabetes for Over 51 Years and Still Kicking

My life with diabetes has been like a roller coaster ride—both exciting and challenging, yet I wouldn't have wanted it any other way! Today, I am sixty-one years young and in good shape, and I have a 2nd degree Black Belt in Tae Kwon Do. I have four amazing kids, three great sons-in-law and a wonderful daughter-in-law, five sweet and funny grandchildren from ten months old all the way up to eleven years old. I love my wife, Jill, and we've been together almost twenty-four years. I've had a great career in the diabetes field both in for-profit and non-profit sectors. My life is going really well, filled with wonderful family and many friends. I continue to practice and pursue the "can do's" of diabetes and life. April 29, 1984 was the most defining day of my life. It taught me to never give up and to always believe in the unbelievable. It also showed me that there is more to our existence than meets the naked eye. My accident injected a wisdom in me that I otherwise might not have had. It has helped me to become a more spiritual person. For that I am thankful.

I continue to live by this adage: "Diabetes—it's just a word, not a sentence!" Fifty-one years ago, life handed me lemons with diabetes; I have successfully made lots and lots of lemonade, and I'll never stop! I'm proud to say that I have had type 1 diabetes for over fifty-one years, and I'm still kicking. Keep smiling and "Winning with Your Diabetes!"

yourdiabeteshealthcoach@comcast.net

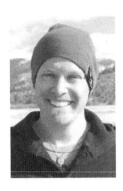

CHAPTER 3   *by Sean Busby*

FINDING HOPE IN UNCOMMON PLACES

From the outside, one would have thought I was "living the dream." It was 2004, I was nineteen years old, and I was competing in the professional snowboarding circuit. I had moved to Steamboat Springs, Colorado where I was training with members of the United States Olympic team, and I was essentially on my own. I had sponsors, I was winning races, and the 2010 Olympics were in sight.

But from a physical standpoint, I was *miserable*.

For reasons unknown to me at the time, I was plagued with excessive thirst and constant vomiting. I was in and out of the doctor's office, each time being told I had a stomach flu.

After being in and out of the hospital for eight days, I realized that all the doctors could do was stabilize me due to my health insurance, which covered me only about fifty miles outside California—where my parents lived. I had no choice but to retreat back to my parents' home and try to get rid of whatever I was suffering from.

It was April, and I'll never forget the drive back to California. I was sitting in the back seat of my parents' car, staring aimlessly out the window as I swung in and out of consciousness. I wondered why I was being put through such torture while my teammates were out training and preparing to head down to the southern hemisphere. They were off to South America for competitions and World Cups, and there I was, headed back to my childhood home—far from any summertime snow.

Until that point in my life, I'd never really spent any time in the hospital. The most troublesome things I had to worry about—other than my snowboarding career—were the occasional pimple and whether some girl liked me. I had spent nineteen years of my life free of any ailments, and all of a sudden, there I was: sick and without an explanation for why my body was suddenly betraying me. It was extremely depressing.

My "sickness" had been plaguing me long before my parents came to shuttle me out to California. Before the eight days in the hospital, it would come and go; I would be overwhelmed with nausea for a few days, and then it would be gone for a week at a time. I also had a hard time waking up in the morning for practice, and many of my coaches and teammates viewed my behavior as lazy. I was still able to compete, but after a race or a long day of practice, I found myself insatiably thirsty. I would go to the local City Market and buy gallon-size jugs of grape juice and drink the entire jug. I credited the warm weather with summer approaching; I was working hard, so it was easy to rationalize.

Once back in Orange County, I made an appointment to see our family practitioner. They ran a number of tests, and we were told to go home—they would call us with the results. When the call came, the nurse said, "Well Sean, I have good news… there's nothing wrong with you!" I was relieved for about two seconds until I remembered how horrible I felt. My parents called a family friend who was a cardiologist, and he encouraged us to request the results and see for ourselves.

I remember sitting with my parents and looking at the charts from my tests; there were flags all over the place—*HIGH, HIGH, HIGH.* Everything was noted as high, and yet I was "fine." We asked a nurse to explain, and with a concerned expression, she alerted a doctor. He called us into his office, sat us down, and said, "I'm sorry Sean, I don't know why you were given the all-clear. But not to worry—I've dealt with plenty of patients with type 2 diabetes in my time."

See, this is the part in the story where I was misdiagnosed.

Presumably because of my age, the doctor jumped to a life-threatening conclusion, yet my family and I had no clue. At the time, I was excited to finally know what was wrong. It sounded like all I had to do was eat healthy and take some pills and supposedly, I would get better. Didn't sound too hard.

But, as we all know, as a person with type 1 diabetes, my body, needed insulin. It needed insulin to sustain my life, and yet I was deprived of that necessary insulin for my survival for three months while I wasted away on my parents' couch.

I remember doing research on the Internet and thinking that I really didn't fit a description of the typical person with type 2 diabetes. Prior to getting sick, I had worked out constantly; I trained for snowboarding every day, and I was in the best shape of my life. But, as I'd been taught, doctors are supposed to know what they're doing, and I should just concentrate on taking the medication and getting better.

I didn't get better.

As the weeks went by, I lost over thirty pounds, and none of my clothes fit me. It was summer in California, and I was wearing sweatpants because that was the only item of clothing that would cling to my emaciated body.

I remember trying to eat and knowing that two hours later, I would be vomiting. This happened so often that I became afraid to eat. Imagine that—a nineteen-year-old man, afraid to eat.

When we asked the doctor why this was happening, he encouraged me to eat more protein. Do you know what I survived on throughout those months? Hot dogs. Without buns. To this day, I can't eat a hot dog and feel right about it.

Eventually, word got out to the snowboarding community that I was still sick at my parents' house. While my teammates began to tire of hearing my excuses, a few of my sponsors actually dropped me from their pro teams, citing they "didn't want to support an athlete who is chronically ill."

I hit an all-time low. It's a huge deal for a professional athlete to lose his sponsored support. The one thing I had devoted my life to was snowboarding; I was unable to do the thing I loved the most, and everyone knew it.

I had actually written a letter—but hadn't sent it—that apologized to everyone in my life, both sponsors and teammates, and announced my resignation from the sport. My plan was to stop snowboarding and focus my life on getting better and finding new activities with which I could bide my time. It didn't feel right to be quitting, but what else could I do?

Finally, in a last-ditch effort to try snowboarding *one more time*, I boarded a plane at John Wayne airport in Orange County and nearly passed out. It was then that I was taken to a teaching hospital at the University of California-Irvine Medical Center and given the correct diagnosis of type 1 diabetes. It was on July 3, 2004—a date that serendipitously also happens to be my mother's birthday.

That first shot of insulin was the most amazing feeling I've ever had. After wasting away for so long, suffering from *ketoacidosis*, I could actually feel life being pumped back into my body. I could feel my body absorbing nutrients. At that moment, I found something I'd lived without for so many months: Hope.

After getting the diabetes rundown from the nurse about my "new life" with type 1, I immediately began researching. That's what I do when presented with the unknown. I got on the computer to find answers to my many questions. There were so many unknowns running through my head. *"Would I be able to eat what I wanted? Would I be able to count the right number of carbohydrates? Would I still be able to snowboard at a professional level?"*

I went to the gym early in the morning every day and did all sorts of exercises and checked my blood sugar constantly to see how my body and insulin reacted to physical activity. I chose to go between four- and five-o'clock in the morning to avoid the crowds because I was so embarrassed about my extremely thin appearance.

Soon thereafter, I came across the website for the Juvenile Diabetes Research Foundation (JDRF) Children's Congress. I read stories of five-year-olds, ten-year-olds, and sixteen-year-olds living with type 1 diabetes. I read how one parent had to go over to her son's friend's house in the middle of the night to check his blood sugar during a sleepover. I never had to do that.

I read how a sixteen-year-old had to explain to his date why he was giving himself a shot with a syringe before dinner. I never had to do that.

There I was, having lived nineteen years free of the disease; I knew what life was like before diabetes. I never had to go through a childhood filled with pinpricks and constant explanations. If those kids could live with diabetes their whole lives, then surely I could live with diabetes for the rest of mine.

Around that time, I also volunteered at a diabetes summer camp called Bearskin Meadows to learn more and to be around others who were just like me. It was amazing. The kids and the other staff there were so helpful. I learned much about how to deal with the "new me," and I'll never forget the time I spent with the campers there who, again, knew life no different with diabetes. To this day, I believe that the camping experience—whether summer, winter, or family-related—is vitally important for anyone living with a chronic condition.

Somehow, after the worst three months of my life, I was feeling grateful for so many inspirational opportunities. I was so inspired by those kids at camp, and by the stories I read from the JDRF Children's Congress, that I vowed to continue snowboarding and eventually got back on the pro tour, competing (and winning) competitions. That's exactly what I did.

But I wanted to give back even more to all those kids who inspired me to keep living and pursuing my dreams despite diabetes. The one thing I could share was the thing I do best: Snowboard.

Thus "Riding On Insulin" was born. I started Riding On Insulin as a program that hosts ski and snowboard camps for kids and teens living with type 1 diabetes. Initially, I worked with established diabetes groups around the U.S. They would set up the camp and pull in the kids, and I would come in to oversee the logistics of the day. It was amazing to teach kids the sport I love while learning tips and tricks from them on how to manage this new disease I was living with.

At one point, after hosting a few camps, a woman named Michelle Alswager contacted me from Wisconsin. Her son, Jesse, had type 1 diabetes and had always wanted to learn how to snowboard; she was interested in bringing a camp to the greater Madison area. With Michelle's help, the Wisconsin camp happened in 2005, and I finally met Jesse. It didn't take long for me to feel a special bond with him. Each year, I would return to Wisconsin for that camp, knowing that Jesse and Michelle would be there. Between camps, Jesse and I would talk on the phone about school and his girlfriends. He became like a little brother.

After continuing to compete and pursue a life as a professional snowboarder, I began to consider how the need for health insurance would affect my current trajectory. I knew health insurance would be hard to come by once I couldn't be on my parents' plan. I also knew that I needed a job that would include health insurance, and that earning a bachelor's degree would give me an edge in the job market.

With encouragement from my parents, I enrolled at the University of Utah in 2006 to pursue a Bachelor's of Science degree in health promotion and education, with an emphasis on diabetes. With Park City only thirty minutes away, I was training in my spare time with the Park City Snowboard Team, competing when I was able and riding often.

About this same time, I was getting burnt out on snowboard racing—a sport I loved. The competitions were monotonous, and I began getting tired of the same old thing. Slowly, I began to switch to a new twist on the sport: backcountry snowboarding and snowboard mountaineering. I was hooked. Being in the backcountry—away from tourists and groomed resort runs—made me remember why I first fell in love with snowboarding. I enrolled in avalanche education courses and I took an expedition to New Zealand in 2007. I loved the backcountry scene there. I remember climbing to the top of mountains with my own two legs and feeling a sense of true accomplishment. I also found a spiritual pull to the backcountry because out there, I felt closer to my older brother, Jamie—who had passed away when I was sixteen years old.

Nearing my graduation in 2008, I came across a boarding school in central Utah that needed a director for their ski and snow programs. It couldn't have been a better fit, and as luck would have it, the school wanted to hire me even before I'd graduated. I was hired as their Director of Health Promotion, in addition to the director of their ski and snowboard program and their head soccer coach.

Best of all? I would have health insurance.

With a degree under my belt and a new job nearly two hours from Park City, I put my competitions and Riding On Insulin on hold to try my hand at a career. Lucky for me, that job "required" me to snowboard with kids five days a week and to travel with the school's competition snowboard team to races on the weekends. Admittedly, it was a pretty *sweet* gig. (No pun intended.)

In 2008, I received the opportunity of a lifetime. A group of my mountaineering buddies were taking an epic, month-long expedition to Antarctica, and there was room for me on the boat. Going there was something I had always wanted to do—penguins are my favorite animal, and the opportunity to snowboard with them was simply too sweet to resist.

That trip solidified my future in the sport. My passion was no longer on the boardercross snowboarding track but rather out in the great unknown. I trained extremely hard to get in shape and get my diabetes under control before that trip. I had to educate all my teammates on the trip about my diabetes and how we would manage when we were hundreds of miles from help. My sponsors rallied around the opportunity and helped me get special tools to protect my insulin, glucose, glucose meter, insulin pump, and other life-saving diabetes necessities while snowboarding in the most remote continent in the world.

Snowboarding with penguins was incredible. We climbed up unclimbed peaks and got to name them, and snowboarding down was even more amazing. On that first trip, my blood sugars were in the best shape of my life. Curiously, when I took the same trip to Antarctica in 2009, I struggled a lot more to keep my blood sugar levels within my target range; it was a great lesson that we never really know how our blood sugars will react to certain environments.

With Antarctica, New Zealand, and Patagonia checked off my list, and a stable job under my belt, life finally seemed to resemble normal again. Then in early 2010, I received a phone call that changed my life forever.

On Wednesday, February 3, 2010, Sandy—a friend of mine through Michelle Alswager—called me in tears to tell me that Jesse, the thirteen-year-old "little brother" from Wisconsin, had passed away from complications with diabetes.

Complications? With diabetes?

I dropped to my knees in shock and stared at the phone. I was consumed with grief and booked a flight to Wisconsin that Sunday to be with Michelle and her family. I replayed that phone call over and over in my mind and wondered incessantly why such an incredibly positive advocate for diabetes, at such a young age, could be taken from this world by a disease.

When Michelle asked me to deliver the eulogy as Jesse's funeral, I didn't think twice before accepting the role. I was amazed—as someone who usually takes forever to write a mere paragraph—that the words of my speech for Jesse came with ease.

That Monday, I prayed to Jesse to give me strength to deliver the words to the overflowing crowd at the church. At the podium, I talked about how I met him, and how he—like many kids during that rough time in my life—inspired me to continue snowboarding and living my life the way I wanted, despite diabetes. But, as I said, Jesse was special. He was like my little brother, and I truly believe that he came into my life to turn it around. He made such an impact in my life that he was, and always will be, my guardian angel.

I concluded by saying this:

Looking at the bigger picture, this is what Jesse would want, at least from me: To keep on showing kids (and adults) across the world that type 1 diabetes shouldn't limit what you're able to do in life. Jesse has enabled all of us to live on in his spirit, and he will now always be our copilot. I live my life by a new motto: "What would Jesse do?" Whenever I have doubt about diabetes, I think about what Jesse would do and what the bigger picture is all about. He inspired me and saved my life.

I vowed publicly to restart Riding On Insulin. After two years on hiatus, I knew Jesse would have wanted me to continue providing kids with that social outlet that he loved the most. Somehow—despite the fact that I now had a full-time job and numerous miscellaneous commitments—I would find a way to host camps again. Little did I know that the answer to that dilemma was sitting in the pew right behind me.

Michelle introduced me to all of her friends after the funeral before we left the church. I couldn't tell you anything about any of them except for one: Her name was Mollie.

I'm not sure if you could call it love at first sight, but there was something about her that caught my eye. I felt compelled to talk to that girl, and I got my chance that night. Michelle's friends and family gathered for a casual dinner to reminisce about Jesse. Mollie was there, and I made sure we had a chance to talk. She told me about her life as the style editor of the magazine Michelle worked for, about her degrees from the University of Wisconsin, Madison; it was small talk, but there was something special between us. Somehow, during such a sad time in my life, I was finding again that thing it seemed I'd lost—this time through Mollie.

I found Hope.

The next night, over Chinese food at Michelle's house, Mollie told me how she had signed up to ride 105 miles on a road bike in Death Valley to raise $3,000 for diabetes. Before I knew it, I was signed up to ride, too.

On my last night in town, Mollie held a benefit for Michelle's family at a local restaurant in Madison. After watching her for hours at the front door collecting donations, the flow of patrons slowed around 11 p.m., and I took the opportunity to sit down with her over a beer. We talked about everything—family, religion, college, snowboarding. When she told me she'd never seen Utah before, I invited her for a visit, and the rest—as they say—is history.

After five months of long-distance dating, Mollie moved from Wisconsin to live with me in Utah. By Christmas 2010, I asked her father for her hand in marriage, and in March 2011, during a ski expedition to Iceland, I proposed to her at Godafoss—Waterfall of the Gods. As you probably guessed, she said yes, and we were married in September, 2011 in her hometown of Waupaca, Wisconsin.

But perhaps one of the most profound impacts Mollie has had in my life is the leadership she's shown in getting Riding On Insulin started again. After incorporating Riding On Insulin in December 2010, we co-hosted the first Riding On Insulin camp since 2007 in Park City with a locally based diabetes organization. Mere days afterward, Mollie was convinced we needed to add two more camps to our roster, and she began planning for a Wisconsin camp in early January and a Colorado camp in mid-April. Both camps went off without a hitch, and it became clear to us that the interest for ski and snowboard camps never died—in fact, the demand was growing. By mid-summer, we received word from the IRS that our application to become a 501(c)(3) nonprofit organization was approved.

Today, Mollie serves as the Executive Director while I serve on the Board of Directors for Riding On Insulin, and we work with kids at every camp, teaching them the sport that has kept me going all my life.

Riding on Insulin has become a traveling program where local kids and teens, ages seven to seventeen, who are living with type 1 diabetes, can share tips in managing diabetes where altitude, humidity, and climate all play a role. Siblings are also invited to participate because diabetes is truly a family effort; everyone has a role. We call anyone who doesn't have type 1, a "type 3"—a loved one or supporter of those with type 1.

Riding On Insulin provides a safe environment with volunteer doctors and nurses on hand for kids to try a winter sport, perfect their skills, and make new friends who are just like them. Kids are divided into groups by ability level. Volunteer coaches come out as role models for the day (many also have type 1 diabetes), and they ride with designated groups, as do I. For first-time skiers or riders, it's a place to learn how to ski or snowboard. More advanced riders focus on improvement with the added benefit of managing diabetes. We even have a mascot with type 1: his name is "SLIN" (like inSuLIN), and he's a yeti. (For more information about Riding On Insulin, please see the website listed at the conclusion of this chapter.)

Our camps are held all over the United States in Utah, Colorado, Massachusetts, and Oregon, in addition to Canada, New Zealand and Australia. Plans for 2013 include expanding to five more locations throughout the United States, as well as a camp at an indoor slope in the United Kingdom. Each time we have a camp, it renews my fire and reminds me of how grateful I am to have lived nineteen years free of the disease, and how much I admire those incredibly strong, perseverant kids who come to camp.

Perhaps the best part is to hear directly from parents how much of an impact Riding On Insulin has made on their son or daughter's life. One of my favorite testimonials is from Bill and Stephanie, parents at our Oregon camp in 2011. They wrote this in an email:

Sean and Mollie: We pray that your mission in life blesses you and everyone you come in contact with … Never quit. Do not over burden yourselves. Ask for help. My Riley has already grown stronger in his diabetes because of you. One day when he is old, and reaches out to a kid who just was diagnosed with type 1 diabetes, his memory will take him back to a weekend on Mount Hood. He will remember that as the first time somebody showed him that he is not alone in this world. He will remember Sean checking his glucose around others and a bunny hill where he took his first ride. He will see kids, like him, happy. You have given us back our son whom we "lost" after he was diagnosed in late September, 2011. Thank you so much for strengthening Riley.

During the dinner banquet at each camp, I tell kids that I like to view diabetes as a best friend. Just as a best friend is always there for me, so is diabetes, until a cure is found. If we treat our best friend with respect, check blood sugars, and manage as best we can, we can do the things we love to do with our best friend at our side. In those occasional arguments (the days when diabetes gives us a hard time), I do my best to make amends with my best friend so I can do what I love to do. The kids think: "*I can do that,*" and the parents think: "*My kid can do that.*" It's a win - win for the whole family.

I also conclude my presentation by showing a photo slideshow with snapshots from the various snowboard expeditions I've taken with diabetes. I've been on countless trips—you'd probably have to check my passport to get an accurate count! Some of my favorite expeditions since my diagnosis include various places throughout the continental U.S. and Alaska, Antarctica (twice), Patagonia, Argentina, mainland Australia and Tasmania, New Zealand, Iceland, Romania, Bulgaria, and Canada (Newfoundland and the Yukon). Upcoming expeditions for 2013 and beyond include Greenland, Nepal, Morocco, Bosnia, and more. I have a laundry list of places I want to go to snowboard, and that list keeps growing. To follow my expedition adventures, visit www.powderlines. com.

When I look back on my life, I truly believe that diabetes came into my life for a reason. Before diabetes, my head was way up in the clouds; I didn't have any ambition for education, and I had no intention of "giving back" to others. I think the diagnosis really gave me drive and purpose to push myself to my physical limits. When I was racing, the scene was always the same—travel, compete, repeat. There was really never any time to explore the culture or the surrounding mountains during the travel part, and it just became mundane. In the backcountry, it's more real—real consequences, real mountains, earning your turns—everything about it. I can dig into my soul when I'm out there, and I know without a doubt that I'm in the right place. Also, I can travel the world and embrace it. Even when I am at home in Utah, I can appreciate the beauty of the mountains in my own backyard while others wait in lift lines and observe from a controlled environment.

In addition to getting my fill of expeditions and travel, I am so glad I'm able to see kids on skis or a snowboard having that time of freedom from their disease. At camp, they can actually be a kid first, not a "diabetic" first. Knowing that those kids and teens are able to have a sense of normalcy in their lives—as well as seeing their smiles all day long—that's the best feeling in the world!

I live for those kids.

I live for the feeling I get on a snowboard in the backcountry.

I live for my beautiful wife who supports me through everything.

With those three things, I am happy, and I have what I need: Hope.

www.ridingoninsulin.org

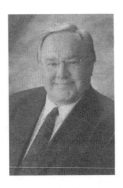

CHAPTER 4   *by R. Keith Campbell, RPh, CDE, FASHP, FAPhA, FAADE*

Diabetes: It Is Yours From Now On; Take Care Of It

I know it sounds crazy, but having diabetes has been a wonderful learning experience and a positive journey for me for nearly sixty-three years. It seems like only yesterday that I was at a family reunion and feeling a bit nauseated, very thirsty, hungry and running to the bathroom to urinate. I felt tired but was ravenous and ate two loaves of homemade bread by myself. I then went to the kitchen sink and pulled the sprayer out and drank from the nozzle. Next, I ran to the bathroom and urinated, and the process cycled again and again. My father observed my behavior and asked me if everything was okay. On the way home, he said I should go to our doctor since he thought I might have the symptoms of diabetes. My dad was kind, caring, sensitive, and very smart for a man who went to night school to get his 8th grade diploma.

Dr. Taylor had me urinate in a jar; he took five drops, added it to ten drops of water in a test tube, and dropped in a tablet of Clinitest™. It about exploded. He looked up and told my parents and me that I had diabetes. He said it was my lucky day since a new young physician who specialized in diabetes had recently opened a practice. By then, I was feeling quite sick, but we jumped into the car and went to Dr. O. Charles Olson's office in a medical building. He took some blood from my arm, had it tested, and confirmed that I had Juvenile Diabetes. He began pouring water into me and gave me my first shot of Regular insulin. It is strange that they did not put me in the hospital, but Dr. Olson thought that if I tested my urine for sugar and *ketones* often, I could get my diabetes in control at home. He taught my parents how to give me injections of insulin four times a day. We were sent home and started the adventure of living with diabetes.

My feelings were jumping all over the place—from anxiety, to confusion, to excitement about learning how to manage my "sugars." Dr. Olson insisted that I attend the next diabetes education program that he offered. My dad and/ or mom went with me for the four-hour daily, five-day program. There were five of us in the class, and I was the youngest. We learned about managing what Dr. Joslin, of the famous Joslin Clinic in Boston, Massachusetts called the three-horse diabetic chariot: insulin, exercise, and diet. If a person with diabetes wanted to be healthy, s/he should control the reins of the chariot pulled by the three steeds. A few months later, he taught another course, and I took the bus to the clinic. It was another new experience for me. I stayed on an insulin regimen of three to four shots a day for several weeks. We learned how to boil the glass syringe and its plunger in distilled water to reduce mineral deposits. The glass syringe was kept in a large test tube with cotton at the bottom of the tube, and it was filled with 91% Isopropyl alcohol. It is hard to believe, but at that time, we used 22-gauge needles that were one inch long, and we inserted them only half way when the injection took place. My dad would inject me in the arms mostly. There was a lot of bleeding at the injection sites. A few scary dramatic insulin reactions occurred each week, and I quickly learned to eat fast-acting sugars if I began to sweat, feel confused or weak, or felt a body part become numb.

Dr. Olson covered diabetes topics in depth, even though I was a kid. I was fascinated about nutrition and the fact that there were fats, proteins, and carbohydrates. He went over the Exchange System of nutrition management for diabetes in great detail. I was given a book that explained diabetes and also had recipes for those of us with diabetes. After several weeks, I was started on a long-acting insulin with the promise that I could reduce my injections from three or four to one each day. I tried NPH insulin but got a rash at the injection site. I was then put on Globin Zinc insulin and took one shot a day, quickly learning to adapt my life to when that insulin peaked. We were a pretty poor family, but my dad would give me a nickel for each shot I took; if it really hurt or bled, then I would get a dime. I soon had a large jar filled with coins. Six months after being diagnosed, Dr. Olson and my dad decided it was time for me to give myself my own shots. They both used the quick technique of just jabbing it in, but I much preferred a slow method whereby I put the needle on my skin (usually on my legs) and with slight pressure pushed the needle in. We had a device to sharpen the needles, and I quickly learned to make sure the needles were sharpened properly. I tested my urine several times each day and would be so proud when my urine was free of sugar. None of my grade school teachers understood diabetes and were concerned about having me in their class. But by the time I was nine years old, I had learned quite a bit about healthcare, the healthcare system, and the treatment of diabetes. I knew how to give shots, sterilize and sharpen needles, prepare a syringe, and fix and select foods that did not raise my blood sugars. When I was having a *hypoglycemic* reaction, I knew how to quickly raise my blood sugars. I was so lucky, just as Dr. Taylor had said, to be treated by Dr. Olson. His training was unique, since he was one of the few physicians at the time who believed that a kid with diabetes should try to avoid high blood sugars.

Dr. Olson's classes left a very strong impression on me throughout my life. He did mention that complications of diabetes were basically inevitable. I was told that I would probably be blind by the time I was thirty years old, and I would probably be dead by age forty. He said that diabetes could impair blood flow to my feet and that I should be especially careful to examine my feet each day, avoid athlete's foot, and cut my toenails carefully and properly. I was told to carefully break in new shoes and not get blisters or corns or calluses. I heard him tell one of the adult men that it was common for men with diabetes to develop problems with the ability to have sex. I did not understand that statement at the time, but for some reason it was etched into my brain and has affected my behavior to this day. "Use it or lose it" became a motto to follow. Other complications were explained that related to heart and kidney disease, nerve damage, gut problems, irritability when blood sugars were low, and eye disease. It was fascinating, and it and would lead my family to often discuss the body, physiology, anatomy, and the impact of diabetes. Dr. Olson even warned us that my older brother might feel deprived because my needs required so much attention. I felt deprived only because I could not drink soda. I figured out, though, that I could get some Hires root beer extract and pour a tiny bit into a glass of ice water and drink it.

My dad sat me down one day and asked how I was dealing with having diabetes. I told him that it was a bit scary, but I thought I was doing fine. He told me he was proud of me for learning about diabetes and how to take care of it. He also said that I would live with diabetes for the rest of my life and that I should learn as much as I could about it to manage it better. He told me that it was time for me to realize this: "DIABETES: IT IS YOURS FROM NOW ON; TAKE CARE OF IT YOURSELF." He no longer gave me the shots, but if I got sick, he was there to watch over me just to make sure I did not go into *ketoacidosis*.

My mother was a teacher and then a social worker. She had a huge caseload and would come home every night with stories that entertained all of us. She and my dad both loved to help others, and we always had people in need staying at our home. My mother had a bit of a hard time accepting the fact that I had diabetes. She felt worried and concerned that I would have a low blood sugar reaction. She also felt a bit guilty since there were people on her side of the family who had diabetes. She was a bit of what we now call a "Helicopter Mother." She wanted to hover over me and show her concern. My dad was more in the background, observing and encouraging me.

After I became a diabetes educator, I often told the story of the 49-cent turkey dinner at Woolworth's. It was a major breakthrough in my attitude about my diabetes, taking care of it, and learning from what my dad had taught me. It was in the first year of my having diabetes. My mother and I were shopping in downtown Spokane, Washington just before Christmas. It was time for dinner, and we went to Woolworth's—a dime store that had offered a food counter where one would stand behind people who were almost finished eating and take their place when they got up. Woolworth's had a 49-cent turkey dinner special. We were excited to get a seat, but we were not able to sit together; there was a person between us. My mother, in a loud voice, ordered each of us the special. She then loudly told the waitress, "My son has diabetes. Please do not put gravy on his potatoes, no butter on the roll, and no cranberries." I was embarrassed because everyone in the store seemed to be watching me as if I were a side show at a carnival. We ate and left. It had started to snow. We were at a red light, and I was holding my mother's hand. I looked up at her and said, "Mother, I never, ever want you to embarrass me again like you just did. I can select what I eat and avoid the cranberries and push the gravy off of the potatoes." She apologized and never again embarrassed me about having diabetes.

Mrs. Skipworth was a different matter. Her son, Gary, was a close friend. It was his birthday, and about fifteen kids were invited to the party for cake and ice cream. Mrs. Skipworth prepared a card table for me with one chair and served me a saltine cracker and a glass of milk. Again, I could have taken a bite or two of that cake, and it would not have been a big deal. I became determined to take care of myself, and I have spent most of my life learning about diabetes, taking care of myself, and trying to not make a big deal out of having or living with diabetes.

Before I started the challenging teen years, I had learned from Dr. Olson and my dad that I could live and thrive with diabetes; that I should be aware of how I was feeling, test frequently, be active—but carry some form of sugar with me in case my blood sugar went low, choose foods that did not spike my sugars, learn about diabetes, and keep up with the latest developments and treatments. I also realized how lucky I was to have a physician who cared and believed that everything that happens to us in life is a learning experience that should be embraced.

The Glorious Teen Years

Testosterone is wonderful stuff. They used to say that "Puberty is a hair-raising experience!" I had attended the diabetes classes and read about hormones and those that impacted my blood sugars. At times, I felt outside of my body observing the changes taking place. My interest in young ladies was rapidly developing as I grew hair all over my body. Acne started to develop, and the frequency of both high and low blood sugars increased. The challenge of managing my diabetes increased, but I had become efficient at knowing what caused my sugars to change. I could give myself correction doses of insulin or exercise when blood sugars ran high and eat when my blood sugar was low. I became an excellent student and, even though I was born without quickness or speed, I participated in sports, especially basketball. I was curious to learn and enjoyed all of the subjects I took, especially science and English composition. People thought I was smart and treated me as if I had a special ability to learn and apply what I learned. I also had inherited a strong work ethic from both of my parents. I mowed lawns, washed and waxed cars, and worked in a body shop at age nine, where I learned how to fix cars and swear. I also helped local farmers during the hay season and lifted bales of hay onto trucks. I always kept some form of rapid acting sugar with me because the lows would come on fast and furiously.

My attention towards intelligent, attractive young ladies seemed to be the main focus of my energies. The young ladies liked me because I projected that I truly liked and respected them. I developed a crush on my homeroom teacher and the middle school French teacher. I saved my money and purchased a car when I was fifteen years old. The men in the body shop helped me work on it, and it became a show car. I was active in many things in high school; I was the class president and a member of the honor society and many other clubs. It was a great time in my life. I wrote a senior project paper on "Skid Row" that got published, and I received a double "A" for that effort. I was undecided about a career choice: social work, English education, science, medicine, or even the car business.

Many people in the diabetes community talked about the terrible teens for diabetes patients, but my experience was not at all traumatic for me. My parents might tell you a different story, though. It was challenging, but by keeping close contact with Dr. Olson and taking charge of my diabetes, I made it through those years relatively unscathed and ready to take on college and to go out and try to make a difference. My high school commencement address was about never giving up, working hard for what you wanted to accomplish, helping others, and making a difference.

Hooray for College Days

I loaded my car and left for the university. I knew only a few people there, and I have to admit that I felt a combination of excitement and fear. I knew I was a good student and had a gift of gab, and I had my routine down to take care of my diabetes. By then, a big breakthrough for insulin users was disposable insulin needles that were smaller (25 gauge) and shorter (half inch). Becton Dickinson later came out with disposable syringes so I no longer needed to boil syringes or sharpen needles. How could something that insignificant be such a big deal? It just was.

My testosterone levels were still raging. Yippee. There were beautiful coeds everywhere. A tragedy occurred in my first week at the university when one of my best friends was shot and killed while home on leave. I had a hard time concentrating, but decided that I should make an extra effort to do well in classes. I was eventually moved to a dorm and had two roommates who were serious students and made sure I studied hard and played hard. I never used drugs or drank to excess; managing my diabetes was enough of a challenge without being doped up. The student cafeteria served a lot of carbohydrates, but thankfully, it was a campus with hills, so I got plenty of exercise. I did not want to embarrass myself with a serious insulin reaction, so I paid close attention to what and how much I ate.

I had a friend from high school in some of my science classes who talked me into visiting his fraternity. The next thing I knew, I was a frat guy going to exchanges with the sorority ladies and loving it. My job at the fraternity was to work in the kitchen and I gained the famous "freshman twenty pounds." Hmmm, maybe that was why I started needing to take more insulin? A week after being in the fraternity, "help week" (or was it "hell week"?) occurred. We were kept up day and night and went through a program to make us into tough and thinking young men. It was especially hard to manage my diabetes, but I made it through. It turned out to be a great experience for me, and I made many lifelong friends who both inspired and helped me. My friend told me that he was going to a talk given by the Dean of the College of Pharmacy about being a pharmacist. I went with him, and my life changed that day when I decided to become a pharmacist.

The pre-pharmacy and pharmacy curriculum was the same as that of the pre-med and other health sciences. It seemed like a great choice. I did well in chemistry, biology, biochemistry, math, the social sciences, and humanities. I was admitted into the College of Pharmacy and really enjoyed learning how medications worked and impacted diseases. I often chose to do term papers on the subject of diabetes and began to develop a reputation of being knowledgeable about diabetes. I was a good student, graduated with honors, and applied to medical school. I was accepted, but when I discussed going to medical school with Dr. Olson, he told me that medicine was going to be run by government groups and he thought I should finish my internship and become a pharmacist. As usual, I followed his advice. I got licensed and was hired in the clinic pharmacy in the doctor's building where Dr. Olson worked. By that time, I was married and the father of a darling daughter. I tried some innovative practice activities like explaining to patients about their medications and how to take and store them. I also developed a unique method of pricing prescriptions using a professional fee instead of a mark-up. I gained respect and notoriety from physicians and soon was doing a weekly drug update for the forty-two doctors in the building.

I had survived the college experience and again learned that I could manage my diabetes by taking charge of it rather than letting it dictate how I was going to live. Needles kept getting smaller, but it was still a challenge to know what was really happening with blood sugars by testing urine. Eli Lilly and Company had developed a product called Tes-Tape® that allowed one to urinate on a small strip of tape and determine by color changes if there was sugar in the urine or not. By then, and after all the courses in physiology and medicine, I realized that urine testing was basically a waste of time since the tests were not very accurate; they were testing the amount of sugar in urine over the past few hours, not at the exact moment of the test. I felt okay most of the time and tested less and less. In the summers, I worked three jobs to pay the tuition and living expenses for my wife and daughter. I guess you can say that the excess testosterone got the best of me, but the overall experience was fantastic.

Professional Career

I was fascinated with my patients' disease states and how I could help them confront and manage their diabetes. Four years after graduation, the Dean of the College of Pharmacy visited me and asked if I would be willing to be appointed to a professor position and develop a clinical pharmacy program. Clinical pharmacy was a new concept whereby pharmacists were trained to be patient-oriented rather than product-oriented. I decided to give it a try for a couple of years, and that was forty-five years ago! I was trained as a clinical pharmacist, helped revamp the curriculum to be patient-oriented, taught five courses, developed continuing education courses, advised students, signed contracts with hospitals to allow our students to go on rounds, did research, and wrote medical articles. I seemed to be good at being a professor, and I have written over 700 papers, some books, and many book chapters. Of course, the main topic of these activities was diabetes, diabetes complications, and new medications and devices to treat diabetes. I also have presented over 1500 lectures to medical groups. Professional groups would ask me to talk about diabetes and the latest developments, and my reputation as a diabetes expert grew. I earned an MBA degree in marketing and marketing research. I progressed from an assistant professor to an associate and then full professor. I am now a Distinguished Professor in Diabetes Care/Pharmacotherapy and, when I die, I guess I will be promoted to "Extinguished Professor." Washington State University honored me with the R. Keith Campbell Endowed Chair in Diabetes Care. I have had a phenomenal career and have become active in many associations, related to both diabetes and pharmacy.

I must have had a high need for recognition, since I always tried to do things well while helping others. I served on the Board of the American Diabetes Association, and they named me Outstanding Healthcare Diabetes Educator in the United States. I was a founding member of the American Association of

Diabetes Educators, and they awarded me the Distinguished Service Award. I also served a term on their Board. The American College of Clinical Pharmacy awarded me the Paul Parker Medal for having a sustained impact on the practice of pharmacy for over twenty-five years. My university honored me with several teaching, advising, and service awards. I was the first recipient of the Outstanding Alumnus Award of the College of Pharmacy. I developed the Academic Support program for the athletic department and was able to consult, do research, and develop a home infusion pump that became very successful. I also served on advisory panels for the Food and Drug Administration and the National Institutes of Health. One of my best learning experiences was to serve on the Board of Trustees of the Diabetes Research and Education Foundation. It was like going to a buffet each day and being able to pick and choose from a wide assortment of activities. My main joy was teaching students and helping them realize that they had great potential if they would think big and always act in the best interests of the patient. I taught pharmacology to nursing students and would always cover the lectures on diabetes and its treatment to the students in medicine, nutrition, nursing, and pharmacy. I could not wait to get up and go to work each day. I was named to editorial boards of many journals, and one of my assignments was to write updates on new treatments for diabetes.

In 1971, I got divorced and was awarded full custody of my two-year-old son and eight-year-old daughter. I was a bachelor father for four years, and then I met and married the love of my life. The major tragedy of my life occurred when she passed away five years ago from a rare smooth muscle cancer of the uterus. How strange that was, since she had never been sick a day in her life, and I was supposed to have died twenty-five years earlier according to the statistics that Dr. Olson had told me. Her name was Patty. I asked her once if she would take a class to learn about diabetes. She said, "NO, it is your disease, and you take care of it." Had she talked to my dad? She was a wise woman. It became a joke at our house. Each birthday or Christmas or Father's Day, she would ask me what I wanted, and I would tell her that I wanted her to learn about diabetes in case something happened to me. She finally said okay, and I set up a short meeting between her and a close physician friend. He told her that she could really help me by never arguing with me since stress increased my blood sugars, always cook the food that I liked, and that I needed exercise—and that the best exercise for me was to have sex at least twice daily. He also told her that I would die if I did not follow the program. He and I had worked out that "lesson" before their meeting. When she came home and I asked her what she had learned, she looked at me with those beautiful twinkling green eyes and said, "You are going to die!" Of course, that was a joke! I never could pull one over on her. Patty and I had a daughter. All of my kids are college graduates and are successful. Remember, you are only as happy as your unhappiest child. I have been blessed.

I stayed in close contact with Dr. Olson, who became a colleague and a friend. When he was dying of prostate cancer, he asked me to present his eulogy. He did not want to suffer any longer, and I told him that he had taught me that everything we face in life is a learning experience and that he should hang in there. He finished a book he was writing and died a year later. It was almost as tough as losing my grandparents, my friend, and my wonderful parents. I learned to cherish those whom I love and to make the effort to spend time with family and friends.

50-Year Medals

When I was around thirty years old, I began to read about the famous Joslin Clinic giving medals to individuals who had lived with diabetes for fifty years. I had always been impressed with the work done at the Joslin Clinic in Boston, and I still had the book given to me soon after I was diagnosed that explained diabetes and the Exchange System diet. Remember that I had been told I would be blind by age thirty and dead by age forty. I remember thinking how great it would be to live more than fifty years with diabetes. I had developed retinopathy and was lucky to get early treatment that saved my vision. I began to think that maybe the statistics I had heard could be overcome. After about fifty-one years of living with diabetes, when I was working on some education programs with physicians at Joslin, one told me that I should fill out the papers and get my medal. I did fill out the application, but was unable to go to Boston to get the medal. It was mailed to me. The medal is impressive to view. I showed my friends and family and put the medal away for safekeeping. I had beaten the odds!

A few years later, Eli Lilly and Company began giving diabetes patients The Lilly Diabetes Journey Award™ if they had lived over fifty years with diabetes. The University of Washington and their famous diabetes specialist and my friend, Dr. Irl Hirsch, hosted the ceremony. Individuals who had lived with diabetes for more than thirty years were recognized, and many people went up on the stage. Next, the forty-year survivors were introduced, and fewer people stood up. The fifty-year survivors were introduced individually, and we went up on the stage. Many were visually impaired, and others were in wheelchairs after a leg amputation, but all of us were happy and proud to have survived. I remember thinking how careful I had been after being educated and motivated by Dr. Olson. Next, a few survivors of sixty or more years of living with diabetes were introduced. I decided that day to try to be a sixty-year survivor of diabetes. It was easy to see that all of the long-term survivors had a positive attitude, many were quite humorous, and each of us wanted to thank our loved ones and healthcare providers for being so supportive. As I write this chapter, I have almost completed sixty-three years of living with diabetes. Dang, it would great to be a seventy-year survivor!

Advances in Diabetes Care

As a person who has lived with diabetes for nearly sixty-three years, I am often asked what the major breakthroughs have been in diabetes during my life. I am glad that insulin had been discovered and that Lilly had developed a process to mass produce it by the time I was diagnosed. So many people were getting diabetes that the world supply of cattle and pig pancreases, from which insulin was made, was getting critically low. Lilly developed insulin that could be made through recombinant DNA technology, and the supply of insulin is no longer a concern. The new method of manufacturing insulin also created purer insulins, and later the development emerged of insulin analogs that worked faster or could last for a full day with few peaks or valleys. We tend to take that for granted today, but it was a huge development for those of us with diabetes.

Next, the development of meters that would allow diabetes patients to self-monitor our own blood glucose was simply a huge breakthrough. In 1978, I was called by the Ames Company and asked to confidentially fly to Chicago and try out a device developed in Japan called a Dextrometer that allowed one to test his/her own blood glucose level. I was excited and agreed. I was met at the gate by two men in trench coats who took me to a room in the hotel at the airport. I signed a confidentiality agreement. I saw the black box, and a lancet was used to poke my finger to get a large drop of blood. The blood was put on a strip, and after 120 seconds the blood was washed off, the strip dried and placed into the black box. My blood glucose value of 143 mg/dL flashed on the screen. I screamed with delight and was told that I was the first person in America with diabetes to try this magic system. Within a year, Ames brought out a meter they called the Glucometer that was promoted to diabetes patients throughout the country. Since I got the Dextrometer, I have never ever gone to bed without testing my blood glucose level. If my blood glucose levels were high, I did not want to bathe my tissues in "syrup" all night long; if they were too low, I did not want to have an insulin reaction in the middle of the night. Soon after that, several other companies launched devices or strips.

Many people would probably NOT remember to put the development of Hemoglobin A1c into the list of major breakthroughs in diabetes care. In my opinion, it should be in the top three or four. It was developed in 1979. Blood could be drawn at any time, and a value would come back to tell the healthcare provider and patient what level of management the patient had achieved over the past three to four months. If the value was too high, adjustments in treatment possibly could lower the value to around 7%.

On February 1, 1979, I decided to be hospitalized for a day and put on a Continuous Infusion Insulin Pump. In my opinion, the insulin pump is another major breakthrough for diabetes patients. I have been wearing the pump every day since then. It has greatly helped me in managing my blood sugars by giving me *basal* insulin continually, and I deliver a *bolus* dose of insulin whenever I eat carbohydrates. I've tried all of the pumps at one time or another. The pumps got smaller, easier to program, integrated with a continuous glucose monitoring system, and now can even recommend how much insulin to use. While on the subject, I have also tried three different continuous glucose monitoring systems. They were great in many ways, but I have developed so much scar tissue with the many years of injections that I had a hard time finding a good spot to insert the sensor. I am anxiously awaiting future models to be developed.

Another advance that may seem silly when you hear about it was the development of sugar-free soda pop. I once drove over fifty miles to a store that carried TAB® (sugar-free cola), so I could drink it without impacting my blood sugars. It was sure better than the Hires root beer extract in ice water that I mixed as a kid. Don't forget the important emphasis placed on trying to prevent heart disease in diabetes patients. "Diabetes Equals Heart Disease" is a banner that I developed for my lectures on diabetes. It was fun for me to explain to physicians, other healthcare providers, and patients that it was so important to manage not only blood glucose levels but also blood pressure, blood fats, and coagulation factors to live effectively with diabetes. I read the world literature about diabetes and cardiac risk factors and concluded many years before it became common practice that it is important to take an aspirin daily as well as a class of drugs called ACE Inhibitors to protect the kidneys. I also was prescribed a statin drug to insure that my blood lipids (fats) were normalized. I spent many years studying whether or not micronutrients (vitamins, minerals and trace elements) should be supplemented daily. I take magnesium since most diabetes patients have low body stores of magnesium. I also take B vitamins, Vitamin C, and Zinc each day along with sustained release alpha lipoic acid. So much more research is needed to really understand the proper amounts of each micronutrient and the impact they have on diabetes and its complications.

The development of diabetes education has also had a major impact on the care of those of us with diabetes. Nurses, nutritionists, pharmacists, social workers, psychologists, physicians and other healthcare providers have become trained to educate and motivate diabetes patients to take charge of their diabetes in order to feel better and avoid complications. We went from just seventeen members, when the American Association of Diabetes Educators started, to now thousands of educators who have a proven record of benefiting outcomes of care in diabetes patients. Diabetes education has been one of my most rewarding activities.

Diabetes has exploded in incidence, and along with it, we have many other devices to help us confront and manage diabetes. In addition, since 1995, we went from having just insulin and sulfonylurea medications to having over thirteen different classes of drugs approved to treat diabetes (mainly type 2). Diabetes is big business. Methods of delivering insulin to patients are improving with insulin pens, insulin pumps, and a new drug that we hope will be on the market soon; the drug is inhaled into the lungs from a very small and efficient device. We are also seeing medications developed to specifically treat the complications of diabetes. It is a great time to have diabetes, confront it, and slam it to the mat. So much research is in development to determine how to prevent type 1 diabetes. I have always tried to manage my diabetes the best that I could just in case a major breakthrough would take place.

What I Have Learned

It is a challenge to successfully manage diabetes. Before blood glucose monitoring and some of the above advances, patients really did not know if they were keeping sugars as close to normal as possible. When blood glucose levels are elevated, or there is a lot of fluctuation in sugars, damage occurs to the small blood vessels throughout the body. Microvascular damage results in eye disorders (retinopathy, glaucoma and cataracts), kidney disease, nerve problems, and a greater risk of developing heart problems, peripheral vascular disease, depression, stroke and skin problems. It thus becomes critical for diabetes patients to be diligent at keeping blood glucose, blood pressure, and blood lipids as close to normal as possible.

I have been lucky, to say the least. Having Dr. Olson's encouragement helped me to keep my blood sugars managed. I also inherited pretty good genes from my mom and dad. I did develop diabetes retinopathy a year or so after I started on the pump. I had a major bleed in my right eye. I was sent to a retinal specialist, and over several months, he treated me with laser photocoagulation that saved my vision. Years later, I started to develop cataracts which I had treated by replacing the lens in my eye. If I eat fatty foods, it takes longer for the food to pass through my gastro-intestinal tract, and I easily get heartburn after I eat. I am eating more prunes to keep my bowels regular. I have volunteered for many clinical trial treatments, and after one heart study, they found a blip; a week later I had quadruple heart by-pass surgery. I was in the hospital for four days, came home for two days, and then went back to work. One of the reasons I have been lucky is that I know the healthcare system, and I see specialists if a problem develops. I was well trained, not only by Dr. Olson, but from all of the thousands of hours of lectures I listened to when I attended scientific diabetes meetings and wrote reviews of the latest in treatments for diabetes. I still have a positive attitude about having diabetes, and I confront each challenge with enthusiasm and a sense of adventure. I often have been charged with not being able to say no. When I look back at my life with diabetes, I see a wild and crazy ride with many successes. I look forward to the next new development, BUT I have learned that "the more we know about diabetes, the more we know that there is much more to know." I encourage you to be curious; learn as much as you can about diabetes. Be positive and passionate. Take charge of your diabetes. Exercise daily, eat intelligently, and take your medications as prescribed. Get involved with diabetes support groups and professional organizations like the American Diabetes Association. Help others and never, ever give up on getting your blood sugars as close to normal as you can. It is your diabetes, so take care of yourself!

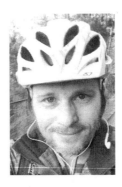

CHAPTER 5   *by Tony Cervati*

Just Keep Choppin'

The Moment

I have always been into space flight, NASA, and all things celestial. When I was a kid, and was asked what I wanted to be when I grew up, I always replied, "An astronaut."

I meant it and believed it.

The best way to get into the Astronaut Corp was to first get some military flight experience. In 1986, when I was a high school junior at the age of seventeen, the Armed Forces came to my school to recruit. I walked straight up to the Marine recruiter and explained that no sales pitch was necessary. I wanted to enlist, get help in paying for college, and fly airplanes.

He was more than happy to get out the paperwork and start going through the process of getting my name on the bottom line. His day was going to be easier than he had anticipated. When he began asking about medical conditions, the Master Sergeant started rattling down the list. I had already received two varsity letters in Track and Field, was fit and active in TONS of sports and activities, and was anxious to sign and start down the future path that I had dreamt about for my whole life.

"Any back injuries, recent broken bones, head injuries?" he asked.

"No, Sir."

"Surgeries?"

"No, Sir."

"Heart conditions, episodes of passing out, seizures?" he continued.

With continued confidence I replied, "Absolutely none, Sir."

"Diabetes?"

"Yes, Sir," I answered cavalierly and without hesitation.

"Uh oh."

"What's the problem, Sir?" I asked while still grinning about the enlistment choice I had made.

"We can't use you, Son," the Master Sgt. responded with concern and disappointment as he closed his folder and ripped up my enlistment form.

"I'm sorry?"

"We can't use you. Good luck."

"What?" I was, literally, in greater shock at hearing those words from the recruiter than I had been when I heard the diabetes diagnosis nine years earlier at the age of eight. I had no idea what diabetes even WAS at that young age.

The life pursuit I had followed, felt, lived, pursued, and dreamed about was just destroyed. I was completely devastated.

It was at the moment the Marine Corp representative said, "We can't use you," that exact moment, that I first truly became aware of the hard fact that, yes, indeed, my life would be completely altered and affected in different ways due to diabetes.

That was the first time in my short life that diabetes actually had stopped me from doing something. The very first time. It would be the very last.

The Beginning

Up to that exchange with the recruiter on campus, diabetes had never really stopped me from doing anything in my life. I raced BMX when I was a young boy, played Pop Warner football, swam at the lake, and played outside with all the neighborhood kids all the time.

People often ask me about my diabetes and my diagnosis date. To be honest, I just don't remember. It was thirty-five years ago, and some of the details got lost. I believe it was in May 1976, and it occurred soon after my parents got divorced and I was just finishing the third grade.

I experienced the normal symptoms such as extreme thirst—I was drinking tons of water—and I began to wet the bed again. After a few days, my mother, who thought I had a urinary tract infection, took me to the pediatrician. After running a few tests, the nurse and doctor came back into the room and told my mother that I had diabetes. I don't remember what my blood glucose level was, but I do remember the staff looking very serious and my mother crying a little bit. Dr. Calderone told my mom that I would be in the hospital for a while, and that was when I began to cry. I had never heard the word *diabetes* before, but for some reason, I remember thinking it was something that very old people got.

"Why do I have it? What's wrong with me? What does this mean?"

The doctor explained that my pancreas wasn't working, that I didn't make insulin anymore, and that my blood sugar was very high. I would need to take shots for the rest of my life. My mom was very upset, and before we left the office for the Paul Kimball Hospital, she asked, "What if kids in school bring in cupcakes for their birthdays?"

Dr. Calderone answered matter of factly, ""Let him eat cake." It didn't dawn on me until decades later just how wise and encouraging those simple words were.

I spent a total of a week or so in the hospital, where I learned about insulin, blood glucose monitoring via urine testing, *ketones*, and how to give injections. I practiced injections on oranges, and medical staff came in and out at all hours of the day and night monitoring my condition.

As you can imagine, the tools available to control diabetes were a lot different during that time period. Blood glucose meters had not been invented yet, nor had insulin pumps, continuous glucose monitors (CGMs), and the like.

Furthermore, there was not an abundance of endocrinologists at the time, and I was cared for completely by my pediatrician, Dr. Calderone, until the day I turned eighteen. After that, I saw another primary care physician, and I didn't have an endocrinologist until after I graduated college.

For glucose testing, a person with diabetes would put a urine sample in a cup, dip in a Glucostix reagent strip, and watch for which color it turned after a certain amount of time. The colors didn't represent numbers; they represented glucose ranges (spilling into the urine): 100 mg/dL to 150mg/dL, 200 mg/dL to 250mg/dL, etc. Same for the Keto-Diastix Reagent Strip that measured *ketones* in the urine.

I was on a regimen of intermediate-acting NPH insulin and fast-acting Beef Regular insulin, and I was taught to deliver so many units of each at certain times of the day and at meals. Since my mother was reluctant to acknowledge the disease, I was largely in charge of my own diabetes management right from the start. By the time I started fourth grade in September of 1976, I was totally self-supportive for the day-to-day care of my diabetes.

Growing Up with Diabetes

Using the tools and technologies that are currently available, it is hard to call my control during my first decade with diabetes "good." I really do not know what type of control I managed during those years. My guess is that, by using a steady NPH dosage and a very narrow range of adjustments for my Regular insulin, it wasn't very good.

Dealing with my diabetes without emotional support at such a young age was very challenging at times. The Internet had not yet been invented, FaceBook was almost twenty years away, and messages were delivered only by the U.S. Postal Service. The support network and communities that we all depend on today were not available then. I didn't meet another person with diabetes until I got into high school. Before that, I wouldn't have known if I were the only one with diabetes on the planet.

I always traveled to the bathroom with my trusted multi-colored glucose sticks and took the couple of minutes required to get a reading. In the fourth grade, I was put into Mr. Roma's classroom because it had a bathroom in it, and that would "make it easier."

There wasn't much talk about my having diabetes among the administration, my teachers, or my classmates. The school nurses did know, but they didn't have juice boxes in their offices or anything like that. *Glucagon* was not available yet. If I was having a low blood sugar reaction, I was sent to the office. I would get orange juice from the lunchroom or be given some cheese and crackers, or something similar, that they could get their hands on. It was a very different time to be dealing with diabetes in school, especially without advocacy and support from endocrinologists, parents, and outside sources.

A few of my classmates would tease me from time to time, especially in elementary school, when they saw me carrying the "sticks" to the bathroom. They joked about how I needed "special assistance" to go to the bathroom, and would say, "don't take too long." They had no idea what they were talking about, and it certainly wasn't directed at my diabetes. They had no idea. Although the teasing probably bothered me at the time, I certainly don't harbor any ill feelings. They were just as uneducated and unaware of the disease as I was.

Another unusual thing, looking back, was that I never carried fast-acting sugars or carbohydrates with me. Not in elementary school, on the playground or bus, not in middle school, and not even in high school during classes. It's so strange to think about that now because that is the first thing I reach for when going out the door. Back then, it never crossed my mind to do so, and no one so many years ago ever advised me to do so. Weird, right? Growing up with diabetes was very different back then.

A lot of time and clinical trials have passed since I was diagnosed, but the goals of diabetes care are still fundamentally the same. The logistics of the treatment of diabetes remain the same, although the technologies are much improved. After 52,000 injections, I switched to insulin pump therapy, and instead of urine testing, I now have used over 85,000 fingersticks to document my blood glucose.

Sports and Movement are the Keys

Once I began high school, my interaction with diabetes began to change drastically. I began playing football in my freshman year and continued to enjoy a successful stint as a sprinter on the track team for the duration of those years.

As I began to play those more intense, organized sports, the technologies I was using to control my diabetes began to change, as well. I became more active and aggressive in my diabetes management. Part of that was due to being active on the fields. I tried to do everything I could to get better and to be the best teammate I could be: training, practice, eating better, lifting weights, etc. What I learned rather quickly was that diabetes was a central part of all that.

In order to excel at those activities, I needed to not only understand as well as possible the basics of diabetes, but also to develop my own personal routines and understanding of how my body responded to exercise with the disease. It was a slow process, for sure, and one that was (and is) ever changing. What worked when I was a freshman at 165 pounds no longer provided the same results two years later and twenty pounds heavier.

When I got to college, my physical activity level dropped off sharply. I still hit the weights a couple of times a week, but I was so tired of running that I just didn't. I had very little in terms of structured aerobic activity for about twelve months. I began to notice that I was running much higher blood sugars, given the same amount of carbohydrates, and I really just felt out of shape. I needed to get myself moving again.

One day while commuting to class, I noticed a sign that read "Grand Opening" outside a retail store that had been empty for some time. I looked to see what the new space was, and it turned out to be a family-owned bike shop. Now, I am not exactly sure what triggered the response in me, but I knew *instantly* that this was the answer I had been looking for.

This was what I was supposed to be doing.

What I was born to do.

I was in the store the next day to buy my very first mountain bike. That purchase began a friendship with the owners, the Yeagers, and I loitered around the shop as often as possible. My bike traveled with me to school frequently, and I began to find myself making time to ride as often as I could: between classes, after school, before lunch, whenever and wherever I could.

I just wanted to ride my bike.

That time proved to be the most pivotal and important of my life with diabetes to that point. I had been very active in all types of sports at all different ages. Even though the technology to manage my diabetes was not "state of the art" through the first years, my health is perfect after thirty-five years of having type 1 diabetes. Not a single inclination of retinopathy, no liver or kidney issues, nothing related to diabetes damage. Exercise and sports have been the key components to maintaining my good health, given the limitations of diabetes care in the mid-1970s.

Team Racing

About a year and a half after graduating from college, I left New Jersey and headed to North Carolina. I quit my job, packed everything in my truck, and headed out. I didn't have a job or destination in mind; I just knew that New Jersey wasn't the place for me.

I landed in Chapel Hill, North Carolina and was taken by the strength and size of the cycling community there. I was immediately at home, finding a large array of friends to ride and train with. I quickly became aware of the local riders' high level of talent. Coupled with the ability to ride outside all year round, I soon was working to get faster and more fit to ride farther on more adventurous routes.

Getting better control over my diabetes was a key to making those goals a reality. I began to really pay attention to my diet and how it affected my blood sugars. My endocrinologist switched my *Lantus*® insulin to split doses and implemented different *bolus* doses for eating during, before, and after riding. After almost twenty years with type 1, I began to slowly learn and understand, more and more, about the interlaced relationship between diabetes and athletic performance, particularly on the bike.

In 2005, a friend of mine registered for a 24-hour mountain bike race. The vast majority of racers who attempt this type of event did it with a team of riders. The idea is to complete as many laps as possible around a specific mountain bike course in the 24-hour time frame. I had never heard of an event like that before, and I was intrigued. I traveled to the event to act as a support person and to witness that type of race.

I was hooked.

A few months later, I signed up for my first mountain bike race: A 24-hour race on a two-person team. I figured it would be fun, and I had no trepidation about attempting it as a person with diabetes. My plan was to simply use less *Lantus*® and eat as regularly as possible.

Right.

As you can imagine, the race was pretty much a grease fire. I ran *hypoglycemic* for nearly fourteen hours. My lap times were the slowest of any racers at the event, and my team finished dead last.

After the race ended, a few of us traveled the three hours home in the car together. Everyone talked about the event and the fun they had riding and camping. I sat in complete silence, staring out the window and watching the road pass by.

Frustrated. Sad. Defeated. Angry. Crying.

It was the same feeling I had had when denied by the recruiter back in high school all those years ago. This time, however, I felt like I had the ability to control the outcome a little more. When the drive was nearly over, I turned to my friends in the car and spoke for the first time. In a very calm, serious, and declarative tone I stated, "I promise all of you: I will successfully complete one of these 24-hour races *solo*. Count on it!"

Getting Organized

One of the first things I needed to do was find an endocrinologist who had experience with patients with diabetes *and* with cycling and endurance athletes. A friend at the gym where I was teaching cycle classes recommended Joe Largy from the University of North Carolina Diabetes Care Center (UNC DCC). Joe had type 1 diabetes, also wore an insulin pump, and did road and mountain cycling. In fact, he had run a study a year earlier with a team of four people with type 1 diabetes in a 24-hour MTB race.

I stood in a line at the Take Control of Your Diabetes (TCOYD) conference in Raleigh, North Carolina, where Joe was giving free diabetes screenings. When it was my time, I went up and introduced myself, asked him to skip the screening, and told him what I wanted to do. He listened and handed me a business card with instructions to call and make an appointment.

After we talked at his office in more detail, he said he didn't know anybody with type 1 who had ever done an event like that before. He was interested in helping and in accumulating data generated by a person with type 1 diabetes over the course of a 24-hour solo event. We began to talk specifics.

He told me that the first thing I needed to do was switch to pump therapy.

My response was absolutely, positively not. No way. Not gonna happen.

Joe explained that it was the only way this was going to happen, or he would be hesitant to pursue this objective with me. We agreed to disagree on that point, and I went home to take some time to think about it.

Although I really didn't want to change my diabetes management, which I viewed as "working," I realized that I needed to accept a new and possibly uncomfortable treatment option to progress to where I wanted to be. I needed to trust Joe's experience and my instincts that this was the way it needed to be to make sure I could obtain my goals. So, in 2005, I agreed to make the change.

After agreeing to switch to an insulin pump, and actually beginning to use one, I was not sure what I was ever concerned about in the first place. It took all of three days to get used to it, and the advantages a modern insulin pump provides are simply immeasurable and invaluable. I should have turned my back on multiple daily injection therapy a long, long time ago.

The Certified Diabetes Educator, Camille, who, by the way, also has type 1 diabetes and is an accomplished runner, taught me how to use the new device. I began to painstakingly record all the details of every training session that Joe and I planned out. During those rides, we modified *basal* rates and ratios, and juggled carbohydrate intakes to figure out what worked best for longer and longer stints in the saddle. It was an eye opening experience to see, really see, the interaction between all the moving parts. With this knowledge and legion of new tools, a whole new world had been opened to me, and I quickly set out to explore all of it.

I began to get a handle on what would happen given a set of circumstances, and I could make adjustments on the spur of the moment given a set of events. My ride times got longer and longer. Before, I would have needed to take in seventy grams of carbohydrates before a ride, but now I could manipulate the pump and intake to allow me to decide last minute to head out on the bike. I increased my ride times from four to six to eight hours with each conversation with Joe and Camille. Soon, ten and twelve hours of riding had gone by. At that point, we knew not only that a 24-hour solo race with type 1 diabetes could be completed, but also how to do it.

With the months of work we had done, doing all of this riding and data collecting, I was nominated for the 2005 LifeScan Prize for Athletic Achievement to be awarded at the Diabetes Exercise and Sports Association (DESA) conference in West Chester, Pennsylvania. Although I didn't win any of the awards, I was invited to attend as an *honorable mention.*

I went to the conference and awards program and listened to the three winners detail their lives with diabetes: the things they had done and what they wanted to accomplish with the proceeds of their winnings. In particular, I was intrigued by the presentation given by a winner from Wales. She spoke at length about a group that she had started whose mission it was to inspire and educate people with diabetes about continuing their outdoor/mountain pursuits.

When I got back to my dorm room on campus that evening, I kept thinking about the work she was doing to help others. I was very moved and inspired to try to help others in the same manner. I struggled with diabetes virtually alone, as a child, and I wanted to change that in some way for others facing the same path.

At 1:15 a.m., the idea of what I wanted to do, what I felt compelled to do, came to me, and I registered the Type1Rider domain. I wasn't sure how to get started, but I had a base from which to someday host my goals. The Type1Rider Organization was hatched.

At first, I began to simply use the website to post simple text entries about my training rides, pump settings, diet, performance, and blood sugars for each of my training rides. I wanted to start sharing it openly, and to make it easier to transfer information to the staff at the UNC DCC, but it quickly began to morph into something else.

Within a few weeks, I got an email from a gentleman on the west coast who had stumbled across my page via a search engine. He also had type 1 diabetes, was training for a Half Ironman triathlon, and asked specific questions about things I wrote about extended stints on the bike. Other emails began to quickly follow from athletes with diabetes from all over the place.

It became clear that, just as Joe and I had discovered months earlier, there was no other documentation of anyone with type 1 diabetes doing this type of training and exercise. There was a need here to better organize and distribute this data to others with this disease who were attempting long endeavors. Type1Rider began to form itself around the ideas of Awareness, Education, Support, and Encouragement.

For the past six years, the site has grown immensely; it documents my life with diabetes, all aspects of it, out loud. It includes real-time blood glucose postings, entries about racing, training rides, events, and general experiences as they relate to and affect my diabetes. (For further information about Type 1Rider, please see the website listed at the conclusion of this chapter.)

In late 2011, I joined Diane Pridmore, a dedicated, passionate, driven mother of a young daughter with type 1 diabetes. With some assistance from others, we formed The Blue Heel Society—an organization all about advocacy and raising awareness for all people and families dealing with all types of diabetes. We called attention to the issue by wearing blue shoes, whether Nike or Louboutin, and talking about it. Openly. No fundraising or money collecting, just a pair of community vehicles to foster open, frank, honest discussions about diabetes.

Solo Racing

On October 16, 2005, after all the months of preparation, education, and training, I attempted to become the first person with type 1 diabetes to complete a 24-hour mountain bike event solo. I had no expectations or place goals; I just wanted to finish and to document that I was still riding at the end of the event—1,440 minutes after it had begun.

I asked a close-knit clan of friends to travel down with me, and I taught them a crash course in diabetes management: fast-acting sugars, temporary *basal* dosing, the location of the spare infusion sets, and the *what-to-do* in case of any problems. I had no idea what to expect; none of us did. I wore an old style continuous glucose monitor (CGM) for the event to allow Joe to see what changes happened over the 24 hours. This was a groundbreaking day for sure.

On October 17, after riding my mountain bike around the clock for twenty-four hours and four minutes, I finished 16th out of 26 riders in the Solo Men's class.

I was not on the podium, but I was on top of the world.

That was the beginning of five years of racing in all different length endurance events at countless venues. It was an endless quest to challenge diabetes to try and stop me, and to prove that it absolutely could not. It gave me the opportunity to kick diabetes in the teeth with every single pedal stroke I took. It was not only addictive but liberating—a way to shed the shackles that diabetes had attempted to place on my life. On my spirit. I have completed over

370 hours of solo endurance racing since that first race, and no matter where I've finished—first, last, or in-between—I've never lost sight of the fact that just finishing was a staunch victory.

The highlight of all of this riding, training, and advocacy work was being nominated in 2009 by the local Trek Bicycles representative, Travis Goodman, to the Gary Fisher / Trek 29er Crew Mountain Bike Race Team. I raced under the colors of that team until it disbanded at the end of 2011. I was beyond honored that Travis and the kind folks at Trek provided me a place with such a fast and well known group of racers. During my time with the 29er Crew, I won the Overall Expert Championship title in a regional 12-Hour Solo race series.

In June of 2011, after almost two years of semi-secret preparation with Joe, Camille, coaches, and nutritionists, I set out as the very first person with diabetes to attempt to complete the 2,750 mile Tour Divide Mountain Bike Route. The Tour Divide starts in Banff, Alberta, Canada and ends in a small villa on the New Mexico/Mexico border called Antelope Wells. It is known and regarded as the longest and toughest mountain bike race in the world, being 96% off road with over 200,000 feet of vertical, desert, snowy passes, 12,000-foot peaks, and only 10% cell phone service; it presents a challenge like no other.

The hardest part of the Tour Divide is the requirement that it be done completely and 100% self-supported. You can receive absolutely no outside assistance; there are no checkpoints or trail markers. You navigate, purify your water, set up your camp, fix your repairs, etc., all on your own. Riders pack all the stuff they will need on their bikes, and they race from end point to end point in either a southerly or northerly direction.

There are no registration fees or entry forms, no prize money or finisher medals. It is truly just a quest to test and measure yourself against the < 200 riders who have raced all the years before. For me, as always, it was not against those other racers or the clock but specifically a contest in defiance of diabetes.

Of course, having type 1 diabetes added specific challenges to the event. The two most easily recognizable challenges were being prepared with enough supplies to deal with possible *hypoglycemic reactions* and carrying all the extra pump and diabetes treatment supplies necessary for what would be, for me, a near thirty-day ride through some of the most remote regions of North America.

Feeling very confident in my preparation, yet scared and nervous about the magnitude of this race for me and for all people with diabetes, I set out on June 28, 2011 at 6:15 a.m. from Banff. As the initial terror and nervousness wore off, and hours in the saddle on day one began to mount up, I began to believe that New Mexico was in my grasp that month. However, that soon turned out not to be the case.

I experienced a very close encounter with a grizzly bear while traveling near the southern edge of Banff National Forest—one of the most densely populated grizzly spots in the world. We stumbled into each other in very close proximity. As I was off the bike and trying to move away, I lost my footing, fell, rolled down a hill, and plunged into a very cold, very fast-moving river below.

I very nearly drowned that day. At a few points, I thought my life was truly over. With the help of some alert guardian angels, I was able to get my very injured self back to shore, get back to my bike, and ride the six or so miles to a remote lodge for assistance.

Although for the first weeks after I started, I considered my attempt a complete and utter failure, the love and support of the Diabetes Online Community began to change my mind. I was reminded by hundreds of others who deal with diabetes every day that the failure would have been in not trying, in not rolling my wheels out of Banff that morning, in not putting the time in to prepare and learn how to deal with diabetes while *en route*.

The parents of children with diabetes, and those like myself who have been dealt the diabetes card, cannot wake up one morning and simply say, "I don't feel like dealing with this today. Maybe tomorrow." It is with those ideals that I will be leaving Banff again a few weeks after writing this chapter—to try again. I have no idea how far I will be able to make it. I feel more mentally prepared for the unknown than I did last year, but it still is 2,750 miles. The point is that all people affected with diabetes in one way or another will get up tomorrow to deal and fight with it the best they can.

The simple act of leaving Banff again will be a gigantic victory, and any distance I can put in past the start at mile zero will just be icing on the cake. Just as it was coming home from the hospital thirty-six hours after a diabetes diagnosis with a dizzying pile of instruments, information, and questions.

Taking the brave, bold steps to face the uncertainty.

Having a plan in place, and being prepared to adjust as required.

Pushing one pedal stroke, or one fingerstick, after another.

At a steady pace.

Continuously.

For a very long time.

That is what is important.

Despite of or Because of

Over the years since diagnosis, especially in the more recent ones, diabetes has been both a hurdle that needed to be overcome and the main catalyst to some extraordinary experiences and relationships that I have enjoyed. It is simultaneously a horrific curse and, oddly, a gateway providing openings to some rather wondrous circumstances.

Now, please don't get me wrong. I detest having diabetes and all of the sinister damage it does to people and their families. It is because of diabetes that my destined path in life changed. I was not "allowed" to chase the dream of being an astronaut. To a large degree, it also probably prevented me from becoming a fireman, police officer, pilot, or other similar professional in one way or another. The disease has caused some scary and extraordinarily hard moments, and it has, at times, strained interpersonal interactions with co-workers, family members, and friends. It is a very complex foe.

I do, however, always try to focus on the positive side of each situation that I am presented with. It is the same with being diagnosed with diabetes. It did allow me to grow up with a better knowledge about my body and to be more attentive to my overall medical well-being. Diabetes encouraged me to take better care of myself, exercise more, and eat a healthier diet. Having type 1 diabetes truly was a catalyst for trying sports and endurance events that I probably never would have dreamed of before. It made me braver and tougher than I ever thought I could be, and it has shown me that I have an inner strength and an obdurate will that I might never have discovered without those added diabetes-related challenges.

I believe that, due to the trajectory that diabetes laid out along my life journey, I discovered an amazing true love, angel, and best friend who was previously only represented in parables. We are together in a single soul that shares two bodies. Every single breath I take contains my love for and dreams with Diane, and this condition of diabetes, that affected us in different ways, is what made our lighted paths cross.

I have learned from diabetes the true appreciation of each and every day: the importance of hugging, the kindness of strangers, the value of life. None of these amazing gifts or insights would have been possible without the disease that I battle with each and every day.

Will I still dance on the rooftop the day a cure is discovered? Yes.

Do I, in the meantime, accept what I have, and try to make the best of it as I wait for that day to occur? Yes. Yes I do.

Diabetes is rare, not only in its complexity but in the fact that it categorically exemplifies a take-home condition. How you take care of yourself, what you eat, how much you exercise, how often you test your blood sugar, etc., dictates the outcome of your long-term health prognosis. Diabetes of all types can affect each afflicted person in a different way under similar scenarios, or affect a specific individual diversely on different days based upon dozens of other factors. The condition is one that is genuinely yours and yours alone. It is unorthodox in that manner.

Quite a few years ago, I heard a young head football coach from Rutgers University speaking at half time. Behind on the scoreboard, Coach Greg Schiano was talking to his players, trying to motivate and focus them to the task at hand.

He yelled to them: "Just keep choppin' wood! Just keep choppin'!"

That phrase immediately brought me chills and made me tear up. It defines exactly what I feel a person with diabetes has to do. All the time. All day. Every day.

I have wholeheartedly adopted that simple expression, and I try to live by it as I navigate through my days with type 1 diabetes.

Endurance bicycle racing is a lot like living with diabetes. You cannot get caught up in the short-term ups and downs of blood sugar spikes, an undesired A1c number, or the piece of birthday cake eaten for dessert. Those will not matter one bit in the long haul.

One needs to focus on being on a steady path of care for the duration. Take one day, one hour, one pedal stroke at a time, and keep working towards the goals of good control and staying healthy. Have a well thought-out plan, but be prepared for the unexpected. Have the knowledge to adapt to unforeseen situations and circumstances, and continue to learn from all experiences. And, above all else...

Just keep choppin'!

www.type1rider.org

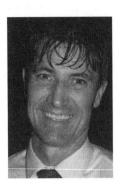

CHAPTER 6 · *by Chris Daniel*

If You Have Diabetes, Now is a Good Time!

There is never a good time to have diabetes, but if you have diabetes, now is a good time!

At the age of three, it was already apparent that my biggest fear was needles. Just thinking about those long silver needles gave me the *willies* and made my knees wobble! My best friend growing up, Scott, always knew that he wanted to become a heart doctor. The more he discussed his plans, the more my fear grew. I discovered that, not only was I terrified of needles, but simply the discussion of blood made me faint. Every time Scott discussed his future, my eyes became hazy and cloudy, then the light headedness would start, followed by my unstable knees, before everything became white and then...BAM! Yep, you guessed it...I was on the floor, passed out! (Similar feelings of a low blood sugar.) After a while, Scott understood that bringing up needles or blood in conversation wasn't a smart move, and for the most part, I was able to avoid those...touchy subjects. You may think I am being a bit dramatic; however, I am not exaggerating! I had serious issues with needles!

Apparently this was a genetic trait passed down lovingly to me by my father. One Sunday morning, leaving services, I noticed an ambulance pulling out of our church parking lot. I was concerned and inquired who was in need of the paramedics. To my surprise, it was my very own father. Apparently, he was in a discussion about a medical treatment of a severe injury, became powerless to that awful feeling, and passed out. Thanks for that awesome trait, Dad!

"The Greatest Adventure is What Lies Ahead" is my life motto with diabetes and with every aspect of life. I have learned that there is always something to strive for, to look forward to, to learn from, to hope for, and to overcome. I am learning and developing to reach my full potential. It is through opposition that our weaknesses become our strengths. Each of us experiences opposition daily; we don't always have the option to pick only pleasant experiences to face in life.

It is through life's challenges that we develop into our personal best. One of my greatest lessons has come from my experience with diabetes; it has taught me that some things we go through in life are simply out of our control. When I received my diabetes diagnosis, like many others, I thought my life would be controlled by diabetes, and I was left with feelings of doom, gloom, and failure for not having the ability to conquer this adventure. It really upset me! As I discussed this with my diabetes care team, they shared their optimistic outlook that a cure was close …"within five years" at the most.

I believe that each of us has been placed on Earth at this particular time for a reason, as part of a bigger plan. This plan has specific obstacles for each of us. Each of these obstacles is for our own learning and growth, and in the end, we become better because of them. Diabetes is one BIG obstacle! I believe that the obstacles we encounter along our life journey are meant to change our outlook and make the best of what we have. "Success" would be defined as enjoying the journey while making lemonade from the sour lemons that life hands us.

Our great planet Earth offers some wonderful experiences. The forces of nature have always been viewed as something to explore. Weather, mountains, extreme temperatures, elevations, water, speed, and high altitudes are just some of the obstacles that I have braved with a "Superman" mindset. I love being outdoors with the ability to overcome the challenges that are thrown at me. It's an amazing moment to look down from atop an 11,749-foot elevation, at Mount Timpanogos, in Utah, after climbing it, and to enjoy the grandeur while you marvel at what you have just accomplished. Or to enjoy a 165-foot rappel off the sheer face cliff at Zion's "Behunin" Canyon, in Utah, realizing what you have just overcome. Diabetes definitely isn't as simple as setting your mind to rappel down a cliff that is so tall that you question if your rope is long enough to get you to the bottom. It is through these extraordinary experiences that I have learned how to conquer the challenges life has thrown at me. What I wasn't expecting was the curveball of diabetes and feeling like my "Superman cape" had been ripped off. I definitely can say that if you have diabetes and are alive today, you truly are still a "Superman" (minus the cape).

Through perseverance and patience, diabetes has taught me that I have to get up and act in order to control my life. If I don't act, I will definitely have to *react* to it controlling me. Each of us, no matter how great the opposition, has the power to act—not just be acted upon. No matter what obstacles we are confronted with, we all have to choose how to respond or deal with it. Ask yourself…"Will I look at this with a positive or negative outlook?" Be an optimist, not a pessimist!

Your attitude will determine your altitude. Having a good attitude always brings you to the top. Look from the highest viewpoint of your current situation. Being an adrenaline-seeking adventurer, I always find that the best things in life are found with the highest altitude, literally, and I have applied that to my mental perspective as well. Diabetes has been a great teacher of this valuable principle, and although none of us stood in line to become a student to such a powerful teacher, we can definitely learn and benefit from it. You can change your outlook from one of doom and gloom to an empowering and inspiring perspective.

In my early teenage years, I was taught that I must limit my sugar intake to prevent the risk of getting diabetes, and getting diabetes meant daily insulin injections. (The truth is, sugar intake really has nothing to do with the cause of type 1 diabetes. The body no longer makes insulin because the body's own immune system attacks and destroys the cells where insulin is made.) The thought that we can cause diabetes by eating/drinking sugar hit me like a brick, and my needle phobia corrected most of my unhealthy childhood food choices. That seemed like the worst thing that could happen, EVER! Boy, if I had only known then what I know now….

Growing up, I actively competed in long distance running, earning school records in cross-country, the mile, and half-mile races. I was even offered a scholarship opportunity with Columbia University in Cross-Country running. I had great hopes for a healthy and active future.

After graduating from high school, I had no idea what I wanted to pursue as a career. The only thing I felt certain about was that I wanted to serve a two-year mission for my church. I was very excited, but I also dreaded the possibility that I would be called to serve in a third-world country, which would require multiple vaccinations. (Yikes, shots!) That slim possibility nearly discouraged me from serving, but after fervently praying, I committed to serve a full-time mission to wherever I was called. I prayed and asked Heavenly Father for a clear vision towards a career to pursue after I completed my mission.

I was called to serve in the London, England Mission. After living there and getting to know the people, I came to love them dearly. I also learned that London is the melting pot of the world. At one time, I was working with and assisting twenty-four individuals, none of whom were from England. Many were fleeing from oppression from their native government or just trying to find a way to face their personal obstacles. At the conclusion of my two-year mission in 1993, I was celebrating my birthday, which is somewhat of a point of interest. I was born on Leap Day (February 29th), so it was my "5¼ birthday." As the birthday cake was presented to me, I remember thinking that there was *no way* I could eat it. The very thought of all that sugar made me sick.

My normal body weight when I left the United States was 179 pounds; however, by the end of the two years, I had dropped to 138 pounds. I justified the weight loss because I was working extremely hard and had not given my body the proper nutrition. So I started juicing and eating fruits and carbohydrates to build me back up. Little did I know that it was the exact opposite of what I needed! Well, it didn't take long before I started having dreams of drinking the Atlantic Ocean and waking up with severe muscle cramps. I was going to the bathroom every two minutes, and the unquenchable thirst became unbearable. I needed answers to my situation and couldn't find them anywhere.

When I headed to the hospital and checked into the Emergency Care Centre, I was placed in the triage room where they prioritize the needs of the patients and treat them in order of urgency. I recall taking a seat next to a gentleman who had his hand completely severed from the wrist. It was wrapped in a towel that was placed in his lap. I remember wanting to pass out at the sight of his situation, and when they prioritized my treatment above his, my heart raced. I felt as though my life was over if my situation was more serious than his. He was in obvious need; I only needed to use the restroom and get a drink! Or so I thought. As you probably guessed, I was diagnosed with type 1 diabetes. Once the nurse who was caring for me had connected me to an insulin drip and brought my blood sugar down, a doctor came in to talk with me. He looked me straight in the face and said, "You have a disease known as diabetes," handed me an insulin pen, and explained that I would be self-administering between five to six shots a day for the rest of my life. The doctor then handed me an orange to practice injections. At that point, I started to laugh hysterically. I couldn't handle the emotional impact of giving myself five to six shots a day for the rest of my life. The doctor watched, not smiling, and waited until I could control myself. Then he stated, "What you have is a chronic disease that will affect you for the remainder of your life." My giggling stopped, and I very soberly realized that this was not a joke; it was my worst nightmare.

Miraculously, I was able to complete my mission and return home to the United States where I started an intensive diabetes education program. Once back in the U.S., my diabetes healthcare team suggested that I switch from multiple daily injections to continuous insulin infusion pump therapy due to my active lifestyle. The thought of going from five to six shots per day to one site insertion every three days was a no-brainer for me. So I went through the nutrition classes that all newly diagnosed patients had to endure. It wasn't easy, struggling through low blood sugars while trying to figure out my insulin needs. Not to mention, going through my *honeymoon phase* (a period when the pancreas starts working again after diagnosis) while trying to regulate my glucose and insulin levels by adding insulin to my body. It was really difficult to predict the amount of insulin needed at that time. It is amazing how extremely dependent on the pancreas our bodies are; when our pancreas decides to go on a permanent vacation, it is life changing.

Starting out, I had the attitude that I would not to be "beaten" by diabetes. So I attempted to pursue previous passions and tried to pick up my talent for distance running. I was miserable. I decided that pursuing cross-country running in college was out of my future due to lack of control of my blood sugars. What a discouragement and frustration that was for me. I really struggled to understand how my now non-functioning pancreas worked and what I would have to do to keep my blood sugars from bottoming out during the strenuous activities that I used to enjoy. My passion for outdoor activities such as water skiing, wakeboarding, hang gliding, and motorcycling was extremely frustrating to me because they all required so much more work and energy to successfully complete. However, I was determined to not let diabetes control my life.

After what seemed like an eternity to obtain control of my blood sugars, I found that I could modify my techniques and be proactive and successful with outdoor activities, especially water skiing and hang gliding. Keep in mind, this all started around twenty years ago; technology has come a very long way. An example of this advancement is the ability to simply disconnect your $6,000 insulin pump from your body while you're active. Back then, the only option while using a pump was to use a fixed needle (canula) still inside of you. Wiping out behind a boat running at 36 mph with a sharp needle lodged inside you is not pleasant and is to be avoided at all costs! I guess if you look at it from a positive perspective, this risk did allow me to become a better athlete. It also meant that I was competing on the water-skiing slalom course with my insulin pump fully attached. I was competing in the field of extremely talented professional water-skiers, while I was competing against myself internally to keep my blood sugars steady. I learned the powerful effect that exercise can have on blood sugars.

Around that time, I started working for IBM. The high demands of that work began taxing my health. I set out to answer the question most of us ask: "What, when, and where is a cure for this difficult disease that we face?" It was during that time that I started to realize that my personal prayer before serving my mission—asking for "a clear vision towards a career to pursue"—had been answered. The real question for me even today is... "who is working on finding the cure?"

My awesome, caring, and inspirational wife, Jennifer, is truly the "success" behind my story. She joined my journey only a year after my diagnosis and has been my hero through it all. She has what I call "type 3" diabetes: she doesn't have diabetes, but through association, love, and devotion is very much affected by the disease. Jennifer and I discovered that, in order to successfully manage "my/our" diabetes, we needed to develop a plan. In one of our family meetings, we quickly realized the need to deal with my low blood sugars because it was really concerning my family. To address this issue, we agreed that if anyone suspected that I had low blood sugar, they would bring it to my attention and I would check to verify. If the reading was *below* 60 mg/dL, then my wife was in charge. She was the Captain, the President, and the CEO. No matter where or when the situation, she was to direct and I was to adhere. If my wife wasn't available, then my children, in age order, were to follow. This plan helped address my personal mindset of "I can push through anything" (being hard-headed) while experiencing a low blood glucose. Having a plan of action and setting some parameters as a family have really helped me down this path and have proven helpful time and time again. This plan provided a safety net to catch me in those trying times with diabetes.

Researching ideas to improve our plan, I started reaching out to others, looking for their ideas and sharing my own. This search led me to the American Diabetes Association (ADA) Exposition Fair. I realized that I was not alone on my journey and saw an industry full of amazing people committed to helping change the course of diabetes. It was overwhelming at first! I just stood there in awe until my daughter, Kennedy, who was also at the fair, started pulling on my arm and said, "Dad, come and check your blood sugar. Please!" Not being interested in testing my sugars, especially in that environment, I quickly declined. Yet she persisted, informing me that they were giving out a butterfly necklace to those who volunteered to try a demonstration with their new alternate-site testing meter. From the look in her eyes, I knew that to continue being "Father of the Year," I needed to try the demonstration. WOW! What a life-changing experience that was for me. The demonstration showed me that I could check my blood sugar in less sensitive areas of my body, like my arm. I didn't even feel the prick. It was an amazing breakthrough for me! It helped me in an area that most of us struggle with—the "ouch" factor, and it helped me be more willing to check my sugars more consistently. From that moment on, I adopted my defining quote: *"There is never a good time to have diabetes, but if you have diabetes, now is a good time!"*

I felt as though I needed to share the news of this great new technology with everyone! It was at that point that my quest truly started to find the best care, or better yet, a cure, for our disease. Realizing that I had a passion for the latest and greatest in diabetes care, I decided to pursue a career in diabetes. As I researched and analyzed companies that were committed to finding a cure—or simply a better life—for those of us affected by diabetes, I realized that my work resume did not reflect the experience that those companies were looking for. This constraint gave me a goal to shoot for: to work for one of those companies and contribute to a better life with—or even a cure for—diabetes.

I left IBM and started working for Diabetes Specialty Center, "Your partner in living well with diabetes," a Durable Medical Equipment company. It wasn't the compensation or benefits that I had with IBM, but it was a great resume builder to help me get to bigger and better things. I volunteered for the next year's ADA "Expo" and spearheaded a new "Kids Zone," a fun place for the participants' children to enjoy. It was a safe environment where they could meet others affected by diabetes, share experiences, even enjoy activities and educational games while their parents educated themselves. Coincidentally, it was a great way for me to network with wonderful companies and to understand the industry more. I believe luck is defined as "When opportunity meets preparedness!"

At the Expo fair, I was able to meet the people from TheraSense, the company that started my quest for what's bigger and better in diabetes. They had an opening in the Las Vegas Territory and, after seeing my passion and drive at the Expo and the accomplishments of my work with the Diabetes Specialty Center, they offered me an interview on Monday for the position. On Saturday before the meeting, I took a break from my preparations for the interview and hopped on my dirt bike to spend a few minutes clearing my mind and enjoying a ride in the hills just down the street. It was one of the simplest trails with the easiest jump that even a beginning rider could manage, yet it got the best of me. On that day I joined the "over the handlebars" club. Without going into great detail, I broke not only my leg but also my collarbone and a few ribs. Yeah, not fun. I do have to say that despite the high cost of ambulances, they definitely did not invest enough money in shock absorbers for the emergency vehicles; that became very clear to me as they transported me painfully off the hill.

After surgery and a lot of plaster, I explained to my doctors how important my interview was, and they released me from the hospital to keep my scheduled interview. Just the sheer fact that I attended the interview was a commanding statement of my dedication to the position. They gave me the job, and I started as a medical device consultant. This position opened many doors, giving me the chance to work directly with providers as well as with patients dealing with diabetes.

Finding myself in a brand new environment, I quickly realized that the best way to communicate good ideas was through end users (those affected by diabetes). Having just had my own bonding experiences with ambulatory services, I knew that the best way to get word to the end users was through the Ambulance and Paramedic community. I learned that in the state of Nevada, each call that ambulances are dispatched to, regardless of whether a person has diabetes or not, requires the Emergency Medical Team to perform a blood sugar check on the patient. The Emergency Medical Teams really loved the benefits of alternate-site testing and quickly became advocates in sharing the discovery.

The community of people with diabetes is a great place to find friends and those who share your interests. I searched for and started attending the local diabetes support groups, where I learned and shared so many ideas with awesome people. I learned many tips on better management, ideas, and recipes, and I kept hearing the success stories that came from diabetes children's camps. I strongly encourage each of you reading this book to reach out and find what local groups or camping opportunities you have, and support them in any way possible. Either by time or resources, you will find the results very rewarding.

Many of the children at camp shared their feelings with me that when you are first diagnosed with diabetes, you feel like you have a big "L" (loser) on your forehead; you just feel different. The kids shared that in school, "you are the one who always gets pulled out of class for the nurse's visit or the doctor appointment or just to check blood sugars before lunch." They shared that they felt like outsiders, and regardless of how hard they tried to fit in, they were different from their classmates. That is the beauty of diabetes camps; everyone is faced with the same challenges and knows exactly what one another is going through. Seeing this with my own eyes, and watching the volunteers who didn't have diabetes take on the "L" because they were the ones who weren't checking sugars, was kind of funny. The experience definitely empowers all attendees.

At camp, everyone truly learns the amazing power of exercise and how it lowers blood sugars naturally without medicines. Sugars are checked at 2 a.m. to be sure that everyone is safe from the feared low blood sugar reactions due to the previous day's vigorous activities and to ensure that they aren't experiencing any "oogey" lows! (The word "oogey" is my made-up name for how you feel while experiencing a low blood sugar! It just seems to fit.)

After becoming involved with the camps, my daughter Kennedy and I escorted thirty children with diabetes to Lake Tahoe for a week-long diabetes camp. After a week filled with memorable activities like canoeing, hiking, swimming, and educational games, we took all the kids back up to Nevada. Kennedy helped by distributing the glucose tablets for low blood sugars, and after we finished, Kennedy asked me if she could check her own blood sugar, out of curiosity. To my horror, the meter showed a reading of 337 mg/dL. My heart nearly stopped. It couldn't be true or happening to my darling daughter. It just seemed so wrong to get diabetes on your way home from volunteering your time at a camp for children with diabetes. Thankfully, common sense came back to me. (The long week in the sun apparently took its toll on my judgment.) I thought she might have some residue on her fingers from the glucose tablets that caused her blood sugar reading to be way off. After washing her hands and rechecking, her sugars came back down to 128 mg/dL. Whew! What a relief. And what a great teaching reminder to make sure your hands are clean before checking sugars.

Reminded of the "five-years-to-a-cure" rumor, I was now in a career and position to see the current status and affairs of emerging products and technologies that companies were developing. I learned about the continuous glucose monitoring (CGM) system technology, with real-time glucose readings updated every five minutes. Now having quality experience in the industry, I researched the company and became very excited at the prospects offered. I confidently pursued my quest of new technologies in diabetes and became a consultant for Medtronic Diabetes. I represented their insulin pumps and CGM systems that were currently approved for use in the U.S. and held high hopes that the company would be able to receive FDA clearance for this "artificial pancreas" device as well. As you look to the advancements in the Biological Medical fields, you will find so many amazing, hopeful, and promising ideas. I continue to look enthusiastically for ideas and companies that are truly focused on changing diabetes permanently and to align myself with them to make a difference.

Diabetes has positively impacted my life and introduced me to some amazing people. I met Chris and Theresa Moore, a husband/wife team who are stellar role models of selfless sacrifice and amazing contributors to those with diabetes. Chris is a Nurse Practitioner, and his wife, Theresa, is a Nurse and Certified Diabetes Educator as well. Together they started the largest support group in Nevada. If it is associated with diabetes and empowering people against the disease, they have their hand in it somewhere and are working to make it a success. Observing their contributions—running diabetes support groups, arranging health fairs, supporting children's diabetes camps, and setting up holiday celebrations, etc.—I found their efforts contagious and invigorating. After analyzing what made this dynamic couple so unique, it hit me: Whatever you decide to do, if you jump in with both feet, you can make a real difference. You can better the lives of others in ways you expect, as well as in ways you don't.

After teaming up on multiple projects, Chris pulled me aside and asked if I would like to be a part of their next empowering project. He introduced me to Charlie Cherry, a world-class podcast producer, and shared their idea of starting a podcast and online support group for diabetes. I loved the idea of taking a diabetes support group online, especially with the ability to reach so many people who might not have strong support systems in their own communities. So I "jumped in with both feet" and joined the team of Theresa Moore (type 1), Charlie Cherry (type 2) and Chris Moore (type 3). We brainstormed our ideas as a team for the best ways to reach out and impact our listeners. The name of Diabetes Power Show came to light, and it really hit the nail on the head. This groundbreaking podcast and audio support group is an amazing resource to empower listeners. Our motto is to help people "live a life full of power, passion, and positive possibilities." Being a part of this team and resource has been a true blessing to my life.

Our team has produced over one hundred Diabetes Power Shows. Millions of people have visited our website over the last six years. Hundreds of thousands have listened to our show through aggregators like iTunes or directly from our site. It truly is a gift that keeps on giving. Looking at what we have accomplished over the past six years, I am thrilled to be a part of helping to shape what the next six years and beyond promise to bring. This is a path that I never would have had without my diagnosis, and one I feel blessed to be a part of.

One of the first shows we titled "The ABC's of Diabetes" (Show #2) covered everything from nutrition to hi-tech tools for management. We then explored topics like "Tips for Holiday Survival" (Show #10) and "Sick Day Management" (Show #14). We got a little more adventurous and learned from experts about traveling with diabetes (Show #9). With the conveniences of modern technology, we have been able to venture to literally all parts of the earth. Each show is about an hour long, and many of our listeners tell us that it is the perfect length to coincide with their workouts (hint, hint). We are able to reach across more borders and continents with Diabetes Power Show than we ever imagined possible.

One of the interviews that really caught my attention was with Lucien Deane-Johns from Australia (Show #51). He is a Dietitian/Diabetes Educator. He shared with us that in their country, the Diabetes Educators have the prescribing power to titrate insulin therapies. What a novel idea…to have the educators, who are actually working closest with patients, titrate their patients' insulin dosing. I am confident that as we continue our idea sharing and online support group, those ideas will take our cause to the next level.

In becoming a successful person with diabetes, I believe that you have to keep a humble approach and learn to listen to people who have walked or are currently walking your path. A few mentors who have helped me shape my life with diabetes include Pediatric Endocrinologist, Dr. Prakasam, from India (Show #48). He shared the concept to "Fight Diabetes…Not your Child or Loved One with Diabetes." It really helped uncover the challenges of guilt and ways that people use guilt to attempt to motivate us to take better care of our disease. In my experience, using guilt just does not work. It may have immediate results, but not the corrections needed for long term success.

Dr. Stephen R. Covey (type 3), the author of the "Seven Habits of Highly Effective People with Diabetes" (Show #69), explained that "we must live our lives in crescendo." How perfect is that advice! The older we are, the greater the impact and energy our efforts need to be. Most people love to be part of a success story but never take the initiative to start that success story. It is my hope that you will look to your own current situation and evaluate what you are doing to better your life and the lives of those around you, and take the initiative to make a difference. (For further information about Diabetes Power Show, please see the website at the conclusion of this chapter.)

The Internet, and some specialized equipment in Charlie's studio, have provided the tools to continue my involvement with the show into the next chapter of my life. My family and I moved to an area with one of the largest populations affected by type 2 diabetes, the southern tip of Texas, South Padre Island. There are leading-edge technology companies committed to changing diabetes, and I personally have found a company that I believe in: Novo Nordisk®. As a Diabetes Care Specialist, I love every day of it. It is awesome to be part of a company that you are excited to work for every day because you know that you can make a difference for others.

Realizing that support groups and camps are very limited in some communities, I took the initiative to start a diabetes camp, and to my pleasant surprise, when sharing my idea and hopes with those around me, a group came together. First, it was my associates at my work; then it was the local groups, school nurses, the local College of Physician Assistant programs, and to top it off for a location, we partnered with the local Boy Scouts of America scout camp. It worked out great. Working with those local groups paid off tremendously for both participants and volunteers.

If you really want to learn more about diabetes, then I challenge you to identify your God-given talent and set out to make a difference within your own circle of influence. When you muster up the energy and zest to make an impact in your community, it really does reflect positively on your own personal blood sugar control. It helps to keep you motivated, especially in the times that you need it most. There really never is a good time to have diabetes, but *if you have diabetes, now is a good time!* I believe in making a positive impact for the diabetes cause and in being part of the greatest adventure. Do you?

www.DiabetesPowerShow.com

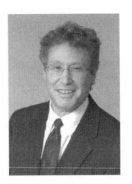

Photo credit by Rick Kopstein

CHAPTER 7   *by Brian D. Graifman, Esq.*

Diabetes: Another Facet of High-Energy, Cheerful, Pressured Guy

I have had type 1.5 diabetes (Latent Autoimmune Diabetes in Adults - LADA) since April 1, 2000, at age forty-five. Well, that's when I was diagnosed—or maybe I should say misdiagnosed—because from the start it was announced as type 2. Either way, the diabetes must have been in effect only a few months before being discovered, because I had had my annual checkup but a few months earlier. And, as almost every symptom of diabetes came upon me, my refrain was the same: "It couldn't be anything because I just had my checkup."

In fact, that prior checkup showed my blood glucose at 112 mg/dL—just slightly above the normal fasting range. That might have caused further inquiry, but nobody reviewed the test results until my diabetes hit full-blown. So that's lesson number one: always follow up on medical appointments and check up on the checkup.

I am a high-energy person, but during those uncontrolled few months, my symptoms included intense fatigue, constant thirst, large intake of liquids, plenty of urinating, infections (one treated by antibiotics), muscle cramps, and as I later realized, weight loss. I kept saying that if I put all these symptoms into a computer, it probably would have found a diagnosis. I had heard of diabetes as a word, but I had no idea what it was.

For those few months, I even developed a bizarre new protocol for commuting: I'd urinate before I got on the train to go home, then again before I got off or just after, and I even started carrying around a cup for use in the car. But the symptoms made at least some sense to me: I had to urinate because I drank so much; I drank so much because I was so thirsty; and I was so thirsty because I urinated so much. That this was circular logic was beside the point.

Eventually, the "I just had a checkup" excuse was getting a tad worn. I started focusing on a date for taking action if my worsening feelings didn't abate. Soon afterwards, someone asked if I had lost weight, and I realized that my clothes were hanging loose and I was wearing my belt tighter, buckling through a previously unused hole. Concerned, I weighed myself and discovered I had lost twenty pounds! Since at full weight I was about 175 pounds to 185 pounds, the loss was more than 10% of my body weight. That was the defining moment: I became alarmed.

The next day I dragged my tired body to work and called my doctor's office to say something was wrong: I had to see him immediately. There, my temperature was 101° F. He suggested that I had either mononucleosis or diabetes. Diabetes? I guess it was when he measured my blood sugar level that my doctor decided it was diabetes and directed me to go to the hospital. I was in New York City, but I lived in the suburbs. I called my then-wife, who suggested that if I was going to be stuck in the hospital, it should be near home. I went right to the Metro North Rail Road and with great trepidation, moving deliberately and labored, I took the lonely trip to the emergency room. At check-in, my blood sugar was 485 mg/dL! I knew I was starting a new chapter, but I had no idea what it would entail.

I also knew that I would approach this challenge with whatever it would take, within reason, because I work very hard and long hours as an attorney. I already had beat cancer some years earlier, through positive changes in diet, vitamins, and exercise (and a little luck). I knew I would attack this experience with the same diligence, dedication, and humor.

Some months later, back at work, I had another scare, at which I can look back now and chuckle. One common symptom of diabetes is blurry vision, and suddenly my view blurred. I went right to the Internet, read about diabetes and blindness, and had a panic attack. Was I losing my sight? How long did I have? Reading things on the Internet can scare the *bejesus* out of you. For reliable information, the website for the American Diabetes Association is a very good resource for facts and explanations. I called my eye doctor. "Don't worry," she told me. My eyes had not shown any retinal damage previously and wouldn't change so suddenly. I went to her, and the eye exam results showed no problems. But with diabetes it's important to have your eyes examined annually. For a blessed week my eyesight actually improved, and for the first time in decades I didn't need glasses! Talk about a fringe benefit from diabetes. Soon enough, my eyesight returned to its normal imperfection. On occasion, I have the impression that my eyesight fluctuates; I suspect that is caused by changes in my blood sugar.

From Pills to Insulin

Nowadays, I'm on the insulin pump with a continuous glucose monitor (CGM), and I have been since the summer of 2010, ten years into having diabetes. At first, though, I was on only *Amaryl*, a pill I considered magical for its tiny size. As my needs adjusted, I added pills and then pill combinations (like *Metformin*).

Eventually, insulin was required, but had I listened to my first endocrinologist, I might be dead by now—not from the diabetes, but from the treatment! This doctor hardly looked me in the eye, and he seemed to want to process and get rid of me as quickly as possible so he could move onto his next chart. He seemed to have a pedantic one-size-fits-all approach. He put me on a large dose (40 units) of once-daily, long-acting insulin, *Lantus*®, and insisted that I wait two hours after eating before I checked my blood sugar, just as it says in the textbooks. Except that the insulin dose made my blood sugar drop so low that I couldn't hold out for two hours. And if I moved around or exercised, my blood sugar level would plummet. Shaking on the subway long before my two-hour wait had expired, I once tested my blood sugar and found it at 35 mg/dL!

I quickly realized that *I* needed to be in control, not my supposed doctor. I started cutting and modifying my dosages, even changing to two shots a day because the one shot daily in the morning waned before twenty-four hours. I had no confidence in this doctor, suspecting that he might be a fake. I switched to another recommended endocrinologist who actually took two and a half hours for my first appointment.

I started using fast-acting insulin, *Humalog*, before eating, with a *basal* dose of *Lantus*®—definitely a big improvement. At first, this was all vials and syringes. Eventually I changed to insulin pens, a quantum-leap improvement. During this period, I had a girlfriend who chastised me for injecting in public, even if it was into my leg under a tablecloth. Finally, I got a new girlfriend—another improvement!

Because I'm relatively thin, my new endocrinologist referred to me as a type 1.5. After ten years of onset, he confirmed that diagnosis by a blood test result when I tested positive for islet cell antibodies. Really? I had been told all along that I had type 2, and nobody had ever said or suggested it could be otherwise. My second endocrinologist believed that, because my symptoms had come on so suddenly and strong, even if it had been recognized during the checkup, it probably would not have made any difference. I didn't learn that until ten years in!

Low Blood Sugar: Sweeten up Sooner Not Later

Prior to using the insulin pump with continuous glucose monitoring, I had more than a few episodes of *hypoglycemia* (low blood sugar). Once, as a divorced father taking my young girls skiing, I was rushing around getting tickets and rentals, and helping them in the lodge. *Schlepping* to the slope, I was repeating phrases and acting confused. My oldest girl, who might have been only eleven or so, urgently asked me if I was okay. I had never really directed her about diabetes, or what to do, but somehow she had the intelligence and common sense to take money from my pocket—I didn't even realize it—run to the lodge, buy a Gatorade®, and have me drink it. Boy, is she smart! She amazed me then, and she does every day, as do her younger sisters.

On another occasion, I was driving locally and knew my blood sugar was low, but I had food at home only a few blocks away. Problem was, I couldn't seem to remember how to get home. After that scare, I made sure to have sweets handy, especially in the car, and if my blood sugar is low, I will delay driving and check myself. Another time I skipped breakfast because I had a dental appointment. Rushing to work afterwards, I knew my blood sugar was low, but I was determined to get to the subway platform first and then eat something. I collapsed crossing the street, just in sight of the subway entrance, but I couldn't get up without collapsing again. Bystanders came to my aid, one with orange juice. I recovered and declined the ambulance that came, but I did determine to get the pump because it had continuous glucose monitoring. The moral here is to test, test, and test your blood sugar and treat appropriately. It's important to review the timing of medications and re-evaluate when you are unusually physically active.

In the spirit of paying it forward, I once had occasion to provide orange juice to another train passenger who had fallen and said he had diabetes. I usually carried candies, meal bars, and glucose tablets, but on this rare occasion, a hot day, I happened to be carrying a small orange juice container. Coming upon the passenger on the platform, that time exiting the Long Island Rail Road at New York's Pennsylvania Station, I gave him my orange juice. Thinking back to my own episode when I was on the receiving end of this gesture, I had this good spiritual feeling, like I was part of some vast overall plan. But I was still in the mood for that orange juice!

I always carry with me two heavy bags, and aside from work papers, keep all sorts of sweets in them. In my main leather bag, in addition to glucose tablets, I have an assortment of granola bars, chocolate bars, mints, sucking candies, and other sweets. There's no rhyme or reason to them; they're haphazard and layered as if awaiting some archeological dig. I kid not. I read a lot, and there are all sorts of papers in my bag too, for the moment I might find myself stuck on a desert island. Recently, before a vacation, my girlfriend importuned me to clean some of it out. I pulled out some articles printed in 2000, and this was in 2012. Yikes, I'd been carrying those around with me for over a decade! Candy anyone?

My Pump, My Fickle Friend

The pump is great—when it works right, which feels like only 80% of the time at best. The biggest problems for me are faulty readings or no reading at all. I also have some design changes I could recommend. For example, give us a button that turns on backlighting from any mode; let me calibrate with a temporary glucose reading so I have at least some reading to go by, for those moments when it's time to calibrate but I'm far from my blood glucose meter (which seems to happen often when I'm way off on a run); and signal when the remaining insulin reservoir units reach the zero mark, as opposed to just when ten and twenty units are left, or when it is really empty, as currently designed.

One day when my pump temporarily signaled "motor error," I wondered what I'd do if it ever stopped working. Actually, my first pump at my training session had failed to work and was replaced before I even used it. So having a non-working pump is not impossible. Nobody told me to prepare for such a moment, but it seemed like a good idea. Thinking back to my vial and syringe days, I called my endocrinologist, got a prescription for syringes, and put some in my bag. More than a year later, my pump started acting seriously erratic, with functions and numbers flying by as if being operated by a ghost. A call to product support said they'd get me a replacement pump by morning. But what of the interim? Luckily, I pulled out the syringes, which did duty until the new pump showed up. Lesson: Always have a backup plan!

One time, late for a fancy black-tie legal event, I needed to change my insulin port, but the old site wouldn't stop bleeding. Blood spurted out—more than I had ever seen from that usually innocuous procedure—and I had to make sure to not get blood on my, and my girlfriend's, fancy wear. Finally, I got the bleeding to stop; it was quite memorable and frustrating at the same time!

I wear my pump on the outside, usually clipped to my belt. I'm open about it, showing people how high-tech I am. More recently, a client who saw my pump showed me that he had one too, although he kept his hidden in his pocket. His pump was a different brand and didn't have CGM. Quite frankly, I find CGM the most important feature of the pump. I'd rather have CGM without a pump than a pump without CGM. Luckily I have both.

My pump emits all sorts of different sounds for different warnings, which then have to be acknowledged and cleared—or it will return to the sound and then make more threatening noises and vibrations. One night at a party I heard the sound my pump gives when my blood sugar is higher or lower than the set range. I picked it up, but the blood sugar level was fine, and the status it was warning about wasn't there, so it didn't need to be cleared. Huh? Turns out it was the pump of the person next to me, with whom we'd been speaking. He had the same unit! Many years back I owned a DeLorean, and nothing was more exciting than coming upon another DeLorean owner on the road. At the party, I had the same feeling when we compared notes about our pumps. My girlfriend peppered him and his wife with questions too. Apparently, we had been starved for information. He had had diabetes much longer than I, and had had the pump longer too. He mentioned the delay in blood sugar readings, something I had never noticed, chalking it up to inaccuracy. Now I see that sometimes the sensor meter reading just takes time to catch up to reality. We exchanged contact information, but somehow I never did follow up, although I've thought about it.

Of course, having all these insertions and devices adds a dimension to my diabetes care. Sometimes I'll carelessly allow the pump to take a plunge—a *bungee pump*—unexpectedly free where I thought it was securely clipped, but with its connected infusion tube still tethered to me! If it's not a complete surprise and I notice it happening, I usually respond with an involuntary "noooooo" while the world moves in slow motion and I view the force of gravity in action.

Sometimes my pump's tube gets caught on things—like doorknobs. And it's usually when I'm moving at high speeds. My girlfriend's apartment has a dishwasher right between the sink and the stove—an area where, as an amateur cook and semi-professional eater, I'm often active. This dishwasher has a horizontal bar as a handle, secured to the stove an inch in from each side. That's a nice hook from either side, and after it caught my tube a few times, we *Brian-proofed* it with some plastic tape, connecting each end of the bar to the stove cover side. That apparently did the trick because I've never since been caught on that handle.

I've been known to take various shortcuts—ones that I would have to emphasize not to try at home, especially unsupervised! Sensors are recommended to last three days, but I've been told they can last—wink, wink— up to six days, a period I've stretched even longer. They can be very fickle, and sometimes they don't go in easily or don't work, at least not right away, or they might work at first but then not. Sometimes the insertion site starts getting funky and uncomfortable. So when I find a good spot for my sensor, one that's fitting comfortably and gets good readings, I tend to want to enjoy the ride and keep it in as long as possible. If it ain't broke, I don't fix it. The same is true for infusion tubes, although they can start to clog if kept in the same area for too long. I was taught to replace an insulin reservoir by changing the whole infusion set and site, although I often replace the reservoir without changing the whole darn thing. I guess someone might change my mind, but for now, if they're working and comfortable, most times I'll keep them in for the long haul.

Exercise: Doin' What I Have to Do

Much of my relationship with diabetes has been about accepting the challenge to better myself. I remember that, after getting diabetes, when my primary doctor said that I had to exercise, I replied that he had already told me that before I got diabetes. He corrected me: "Before, I said you *should* exercise, but now I say you *have to* exercise." That command often chimes in my head as I daily direct myself to activity.

Exercise supercharges whatever insulin I have active in me, so I try to work out first thing in the morning, before injecting any extra insulin, because after I get up in the morning, my blood sugar level rises. It generally hits me late morning, so I'm racing myself in the morning, hurrying to get my fitness regimen finished before my blood sugar gets too high and before I have to counter the rise with any significant insulin infusion. If I dally too much, and have to counter a high reading with insulin, I might suddenly find my blood sugar level falling and have to abandon the whole routine.

Another thing I have to check before taking off to exercise is whether a calibration is coming due. My pump displays the next calibration time, and if I don't calibrate when it asks, the blood sugar reading goes blank until I do. Too many times I've forgotten to check, and in the middle of a run, far from home base, suddenly I'll see the call to calibrate. In such a case, out of desperation, I'll calibrate artificially to the last reading, so at least I have something to go by. But that sets the meter on the wrong course, even when I recalibrate back at home when I'm back with my blood glucose meter. So now I'm lobbying for a way of getting an extension on calibration for the odd occasions when more time is needed.

Not only does it take planning to exercise, but what I take along takes planning. If I go for a run—often on trails in the woods—I have to bring carbohydrates, such as glucose tablets. On occasion, I've mistakenly gone out without them. Once when that happened, with my blood sugar dropping, I ran into a Temple during a Saturday morning service and saw the dessert display being set up in the next room. I told the workers I was on insulin and needed sugar fast; then I gobbled down a bunch of desserts—all in my ruddy running clothes, luckily before the finely-coifed congregation entered. *Oy vey.* Another time, I thought the glucose tablets were in my pocket but was surprised to find they were not. As a result, I almost gate-crashed a kid's outdoor birthday party cake moment, but instead I found a worker who gave me his extra energy bar. He told me he understood my situation because his brother had diabetes. Visions of me harmonizing "Happy Birthday" averted. Now I wear a pouch that I fill with carbohydrates, and I keep a similar bag in my pocket.

Of course, sometimes I crave a sweet not to sweeten up, but as a treat. Since it's hard to find healthful foods, I've been known to bake my own cookies: oatmeal chocolate-chip cookies, made with whole-wheat flour, non-nutritive or artificial sweetener, no-sugar chocolate, cholesterol-free egg mix, and only good-choice ingredients. To keep them from getting crumbly, I keep them in the freezer and eat them frozen (although oddly, they don't feel cold or taste frozen).

I may have a hit on my hands! My girlfriend often eats them one after another until there's none left for me—the person I made them for!

Busy Attorney, Varied Interests, Constant Marathon

I don't run just for exercise—my life has always been a constant marathon, diabetes or not. Professionally, I'm a busy attorney, literally on Wall Street: Litigation Counsel to Gusrae Kaplan Nusbaum PLLC, a boutique law firm specializing in representing brokerage firms and handling business matters, "one of the preeminent securities law firms in the United States." Recently, I had a landmark win at the United States Court of Appeals for the Second Circuit. It ruled that, although the self-regulatory organization that disciplines brokerage firms and brokers, Financial Industry Regulatory Authority, Inc. (FINRA), can impose a disciplinary fine, it can't go to court to collect the disciplinary fines. That was my sixth reversal in a row at that court, the federal appellate court in Manhattan (at least considered by argument date). I've had some history at that court; after law school, I held a very prestigious clerkship there for the recently deceased Honorable Roger J. Miner. At the time, he was being mentioned as a possible nominee for the U.S. Supreme Court but reportedly had too much integrity to tell the politicos in advance how he'd rule on hot-button issues.

I've had success of my own at the U.S. Supreme Court, where I helped knock out part of the Helms Act that restricted indecent material on cable television. I also brought a landmark case to the top court in New York State, the New York Court of Appeals, where it changed the rules for child relocation cases, setting the "best interests of the child" standard.

As you might imagine, deadlines are constantly looming, and projects back up. When things get heated, it's not unusual for me to leave the office several hours past midnight. And the next day, I'm fair game for whatever emergency *du jour* pops up. I also carry work and reading around with me, so work technically never ends. Aside from work, I'm also active in various bar associations and committees, and was just named co-chair of the New York County Lawyer's Association New York State "Supreme Court Committee."

And I'm not just about work and law. I play piano (even sometimes at bar events), and I have written three children's musicals that were performed in the late 1970s. I used to be a recording engineer and record producer, where I produced hundreds of songs. In the past few years, I've written songs for the City Bar shows, some quite humorous. I read music, and I love playing through songbooks, which is greatly fulfilling and a wonderful outlet to reduce stress.

Oh, and I was a semi-finalist in a Funniest Lawyer in New York contest. It started when I attended the City Bar talent shows. I got up with a microphone and said I'd been attending for years, but up to then, exclusively as audience member—"and when I say exclusively, I mean I was the only audience member." And if you think I work hard now, I used to do so even harder, at a large law firm, Skadden Arps, "where I worked for five years—in the space of three and a half years."

I'm blessed to have a loving family, including my brother, sister-in-law, nephew and my amazing parents, who in their late eighties, are still very active. They dance twice a week, my father sings and serves as Sewer Commissioner, and they both enjoy life. Then there's my three young teen daughters, whom by circumstance I don't live with, or even live nearby, but whom I travel to see most weekends, and who make me smile warmly. I love them dearly. And I have a loving sweet girlfriend, a renowned judge in her own right, who is often busy with bar associations and administrative duties, writing articles, and hectic in campaign mode. She also sometimes has to bear the brunt of a not-so-gentle tabloid press, where apparently ignorance of the law is an excuse. She knows music and art, and she constantly amazes me with her intelligence and humor. I've done some dancing in the past, and as soon as things settle down, we're going to take dance lessons—swing and Brazilian samba!

And then there's dealing with life's curves, like losing my younger brother on September 11, 2001 at the World Trade Center. So much of life can be stressful, to say the least. But we do what we have to, with grace and humor.

In Stride, Moving Forward

One more thing about getting diabetes: I don't recall ever lamenting, "Why me?" Rather I took it in stride and put my energies toward moving forward. There's always the constant diabetes care and daily exercise to fit in, and mostly it's figuring out how best to treat myself, even when allowing myself a treat (as I often do).

I read about stem-cell advances with the possibility that my diabetes might become a thing of the past. I've become so comfortable with my diabetes that not having it would be mind-altering. I wonder if I'd take care of myself as well otherwise? I joke about what I would do with myself without diabetes. I'd probably have to get a video game!

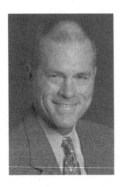

CHAPTER 8 *by John W. Griffin, Jr.*

Diabetes and the Law

There we sat, on June 17, 1997, in our living room. I was thirsty and retrieved yet another glass of water. My wife had noticed this repeated pattern: go to the kitchen then to the bathroom. So I said, "Maybe I have diabetes?"

She laughed and said, "You've been at your sister's house in Massachusetts too long and talking too much about diabetes. John, you're having sympathy symptoms after being with your sister." Both my sister and her youngest daughter have type 1 diabetes, and I had been a volunteer with the American Diabetes Association, so I had *some* knowledge about the disease, but Lynn was not convinced.

Still sensing that something was wrong, I said, "We can easily figure this out; I will go to the drug store to get one of those meters my sister has." Off I went. I brought the meter home, unpacked it, and figured out how to perform a blood sugar check. With Lynn seated across the room and our three young daughters playing upstairs, I pricked my finger and let the drop of blood absorb into the strip; then I waited for the number to appear. And there it was: 486 mg/dL!

"So what?" we thought. But when we researched the meaning of that single number, I said, "Lynn, I have diagnosed myself with diabetes."

"No!" she said. "That's not right!" So we did it again, with a similar result. Again, Lynn said, "John, you don't have diabetes!" I paged my physician, and he called me back. After I read him the results, he ordered me to come into his office the next day at 8 a.m. and not to eat anything until after my appointment.

Strangely, I slept well. When I arrived at his office, the kind physician checked my blood sugar level and promptly said, "Well, you have diabetes, John. There are lots of ways to manage it, so let's get you trained." He gave me some medicine and ordered me to stay off alcohol and big meals for a month. *"This is no big deal,"* I thought. Further reflecting, I decided that this was better than being terminally ill. But from that conversation with my doctor, I knew fully well that diabetes would accompany me for the rest of my life; a cure was far off in the distance.

Diabetes dwells differently in each of the twenty-six million American children and adults who have it. I soon realized that it was much easier for me to manage diabetes than it was for some people, and that had little to do with education, discipline, or socio-economic factors. I saw people with all manner of outcomes: a blind, brilliant forty-year-old lawyer, his sight gone because of chronic high blood sugar levels; a ninety-year-old man who lived complication-free after eighty-six years of diabetes.

The burden that diabetes inflicts is a silent one. Many people, simply because of who they are, suppress diabetes, subconsciously believing that suppressing it will make them feel more "normal." As the years go by, these people are happy, all the while paying little attention to their blood sugar values. But, little by little, the tiniest blood vessels in their kidneys, eyes, and extremities are being destroyed, and so are the larger vessels near the heart.

In 1997, I was a newly diagnosed person, still unafraid of the world and of diabetes. Now I have lived with diabetes for fifteen years, and as a trial lawyer, I know there is nothing I can do about the uniqueness of humanity. Yet the tragedy of bright and passionate people afflicted with amputations, blindness, kidney dialysis, and needless deaths still troubles me to this day.

A burst of energy carried me through nutritional counseling, carbohydrate counting, and blood glucose monitoring. A strange sense of courage kept driving me forward, perhaps from sheer ignorance. After all, many of my healthcare providers repeated the mantra that diabetes can be managed and that those with diabetes can have happy full lives. That was the plan.

Then, over the next several days, a gray pall came over me. Something was wrong. I felt no joy, and I wanted to be alone. While we were visiting my mother-in-law, my wife suggested that I take our three small daughters to one of their favorite places, a bookstore. While they gleefully searched for ways to spend their book money, I wandered down the aisle, looking for books on diabetes.

The girls and I headed back to the house with a bag full of books, and when we arrived, I went to the bedroom and began to explore the diabetes books. As I dove into them, it became apparent to me that the journey of life with diabetes often begins with a path through some depression and anxiety. As my eyes passed over those words, they welled with tears that flowed freely for a few minutes. I could not explain them, but there they were. And I was not alone, and not narcissistic just because of these feelings. I realized that other people have walked this path, and it was okay to feel this way. The pall wasn't lifted, but I was relieved in a way.

Yet a pattern developed over the next few weeks. Many well-meaning friends asked me, "Aren't you glad it's not cancer?" or "Aren't you glad you can control it with diet and medicine and exercise?" I would grimace inside and say, "Of course." But no, I was *not glad* in any sense of the word. And overlaid on that anxiety was pure guilt: the guilt of feeling depressed because of my diagnosis of diabetes. My diabetes isn't terminal cancer, and it is controllable. What kind of person feels sorry for himself when diagnosed with diabetes? Who am I to be depressed when others struggle with much more tragic conditions than mine?

I began to mope around the house, avoiding social situations where I would have to interact with others. One day, my wife insisted we attend a museum opening. "No!" I said. "I don't feel like it." She insisted, so I glumly went with her, knowing that there would be awkward conversation, no wine, and no good food. At the museum, I tried to be invisible, but a neighbor from across the street approached me with the time-honored greeting: "How are you, John?" I looked at her and said, ""Not so good since I can't drink, can't eat good food, and got diagnosed with diabetes." She looked at me, gave me a hug, and said, "John, that's such a drag!" At her remarkable honesty, I burst into tears, thanking her profusely. That encounter changed the trajectory of the journey. It was what it was: guilt or no guilt. Acceptance was important, and from that day forward, there was acceptance.

Yes, diabetes is a scourge some days, and yes, it is manageable, and yes, it is a journey. At the same time, paradoxically, the journey has been full of wonderful encounters and experiences that would never have been possible but for living with diabetes.

The journey took me from managing with diet and medicine, then with diet alone, then with medicines again, and then hearing the dreaded news: "You must go on insulin, John." It was so weird to travel back to that feeling of failure: Other people can do it without insulin, so why can't a successful lawyer do it? Three years after diagnosis, my wife and I sat in our bedroom with the insulin pen dialed up to the proper dose, and once again, as diabetes so often brings about, the tears flowed. It seems paradoxical that insulin, a literal life saver, can cause such grief and feelings of worthlessness, but it did. After being cleansed by the tears, I found the first injection to be easy. After all, I had known many people with type 1 diabetes.

Now insulin is my friend, and I have no clue why I was ever depressed about using the most important item in the tool chest for controlling blood sugar levels. And insulin has many forms and methods to administer it. Those choices include once-a-day insulin, fast-acting insulin, those that peak, and those that don't. In the many years that insulin has been in my life, I have used all of them, and I have used both pens and pumps.

One of my life-altering events was my encounter with another trial lawyer with diabetes, years before I was diagnosed. In 1994, a couple came to my office for a consultation. The husband explained that he had lost his job as a UPS driver because he had diabetes and was ordered to go on insulin or be hospitalized. UPS had a blanket ban on any drivers who managed diabetes with insulin. Of course, I didn't have diabetes, and I knew next to nothing about employment law. I had heard that the Americans With Disabilities Act protected people against this sort of discrimination, so I tried to help him. In so doing, I looked for some sort of non-profit organization dedicated to diabetes, and I found the American Diabetes Association (ADA), which helped me a lot. It turned out that the Association helped fight this sort of discrimination, and I was referred to a volunteer in San Antonio.

The volunteer was a feisty endocrinologist who taught at the medical school, conducted research, and treated patients: a "triple threat," he called himself. The client had no money, but this doctor said, ""Tell him to come to San Antonio, and I will help him for no charge." Here was a world-class endocrinologist, who didn't know me from Adam, who said to tell my client to just drive to San Antonio. I was ecstatic; the client did drive to San Antonio, and then I was summoned to meet with him as well.

Inviting us into his office, the doctor said, in his own salty way, that the UPS ban made no sense, and it kept good people out of jobs that they were perfectly able to do. He would write a report and show the federal judge how wrong and unnecessary that ban was. He felt that people should be judged individually, not lumped into groups. He was brimming with confidence, competence, and compassion for my client. It was almost mystical.

When the federal judge read his report, he ruled in our favor, saying that the time for blanket bans was over. UPS would not let my client drive, but it paid him a good settlement and promoted him into management. Years later, UPS further altered its restrictive policies toward workers with diabetes, but even now, there is work to do to make UPS a better employer for people with diabetes.

All this was pretty good for a small town lawyer who did not have diabetes. Helping people has its own way of making us feel better. I will never forget that young UPS worker in my office. I told him to be sure to monitor his blood sugar to prove that he was well managed. His eyes filled with tears, and he said, "We have a baby, and we can't afford test strips because they cost a dollar per strip." Shocked at such a cost but not moved emotionally, I said that our firm would help with the strips and for him to monitor faithfully, which he did. Now, of course, since I, too, am walking that path, I would weep right along with that client sharing his story. A few months after the successful resolution with UPS, the father of a young college graduate called me when he heard about the UPS worker from fellow volunteers with the American Diabetes Association. His son had type 1 diabetes and was offered a job as a police officer, but when the department discovered that he had diabetes, it revoked the offer. That call began a seven-year journey through the federal courts, and it built a friendship that has lasted to this day.

It was during that seven-year journey that diabetes afflicted me, causing my wife to note that this was taking client empathy too far. Of course, nobody thinks it will take seven years to finish a legal case; the UPS case had sailed to completion in one year. But not this time. Twice the federal judge tossed the police-officer case out of the court system without a trial. Why? Because, as I learned, some courts held that all people with insulin-treated diabetes were dangerous to humanity. The City of San Antonio forbade anyone with insulin-treated diabetes to be police officers, and it took seven long years to win a change in policy. Finally, the nation's second highest court ruled that each person with diabetes should be evaluated individually on his or her own merit. There was a great celebration and a picture of Jeff Kapche and me on the cover of *Diabetes Forecast* magazine. We thought the world had changed.

Well, it had. But I soon learned that just as there were few steps forward in the quest for a cure for diabetes, and for the better treatment of diabetes, these were also only a few steps forward for fair treatment of people with diabetes. A few years later, my hero, Jeff Kapche, gave another seven years of his life to breaking down another blanket ban—this one from the FBI. It banned as Special Agents anyone who managed diabetes by insulin injections. It took a jury trial and an appeal in 2012 to confirm this wall tumbling down. Now, men and women who want to be Special Agents can do so without fear of being banned as they once were. And we have opened even more doors for them, such as with the State Department, which for decades would not hire those with insulin-treated diabetes as Foreign Service Officers. Now the first two are serving—one in the Czech Republic and one in Haiti.

As I served on more and more ADA committees, I learned more about the wonderful work being done by scientists, healthcare professionals, and diabetes advocates. But we also learned more about challenges. We learned that children with diabetes were being rounded up and sent to separate schools, away from their normal schools. We attacked that, and we are winning those battles, but they still present a real challenge. Some people argue that the separate schools are equal to their own schools and that being in a separate school is better for children with diabetes. Some say that children can't take care of their diabetes unless a nurse is there all the time to care for them. Those groups claim that only a nurse can help a child, and if no nurse is present to help a child who needs insulin, then just call an ambulance and hope for the best. Those groups claim that it is a criminal act for a trained volunteer to help a child with insulin. Those groups claim that, despite the fact that 99% of all insulin injections and pump *boluses* are done by trained volunteers, they are not nurses and should not be administering insulin. This stance makes our blood boil, and we have worked with medical groups and the Department of Education to make sure every child gets the care s/he needs, even if a nurse is not on campus. No child in need of insulin should be left to the mercy of an EMS ambulance call and response.

These challenges, along with those surrounding better care and a cure for this disease, empowered me to become more involved with the ADA. Serving as Chair of the National Board of Directors in 2011 allowed me to testify in Congress, seeking funds for a cure and better diabetes treatment and oppose discrimination against our diabetes community. (For further information about the ADA, please see the website at the conclusion of this chapter.)

Yet during those years, I sometimes suppressed diabetes, just like the millions of other people who do this. Shortly before joining the ADA's Executive Committee, my A1c was hovering above 8%. This was a point of embarrassment. If I, a leading diabetes volunteer in this country, could not stay below 7%, how would I ever be a good mentor for others?

So I went to the office of a therapist friend of mine, yearning to find out why this was happening. As the conversation unfolded, I revealed that on Friday nights, diabetes would "disappear" from my life. As the Mexican food and margaritas flowed, the meter stayed put, and I did not get insulin at least until bedtime. My blood sugar values were skewed from those two- to three-hour "diabetes holidays." Of course, eating Mexican food and not injecting insulin was a recipe for very high glucose values and blood sugar management disaster. The rest of each weekend would focus on trying to correct these issues. I told the therapist that, for those hours with my friends, I refused to count tortilla chips and carbohydrates.

He asked, ""Why do you suppose you do that, John?"

I considered that question, then burst into tears: "I just wanted, for one night a week, to be like everybody else." That longing feeling can still make my eyes well with tears, and when I think of small children who just want to be like their peers, I often weep for them as well.

My friend the therapist then asked if I thought I was defeating the disease by blotting it out for those hours. I said that I guessed that was the way I felt. He then asked if I thought that was right. Of course, at that point, I knew it was wrong. There is no "holiday." Each chip does have carbohydrates. And there is no vacation. I would have to understand this and act on it, and I was fortunate to be able to do so. Millions go through the same issues but do not get the help that they need to make friends with the disease and learn to live with it, managing it twenty-four hours a day, seven days a week.

All of this reminds me of something my father used to say: "When you get knocked off the horse, you have get back on, Johnny." That was true for me with my own diabetes as well as for the efforts to reach the ADA's vision: a world free of diabetes and all its burdens. This fifteen-year journey, paradoxically, is one of the most rewarding things to have happened to me in my life. The relationships, the children's smiles, the victories, the young researcher getting her first ADA grant, the walls of exclusion being torn down—all of this has been precious.

Nobody would wish diabetes on a worst enemy, but today I can honestly say that it has been a great thing to happen. In terms of health, diet, weight, friendships, and the determination to make a difference and to stay on top of the law and medicine, having and living with diabetes has made me a more productive person with an optimistic view of life and this disease. For now, we live with it, even as we happily charge forward to help improve the lives of the twenty-six million American children and adults with diabetes. And in that, we can consider ourselves privileged!

www.diabetes.org   (American Diabetes Association)

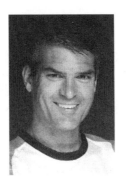

Photo credit by Josh Norris

CHAPTER 9   *by Jay Hewitt*

What is Your Finish Line?

My name was not on the list. I was a fifteen-year-old sophomore in high school, standing alone in the lobby of the gymnasium at J.L. Mann High School in Greenville, South Carolina, staring at the sheet of paper pinned to the corkboard behind the glass. I had been cut from the junior varsity basketball team. I was devastated. I had that sinking feeling in the pit of my stomach. What do I do now?

Looking back years later, I now realize that it was a significant point in my life. How would I respond to adversity? To an obstacle? To rejection, failure? Do I give up, embittered and dejected, feeling sorry for myself? Do I blame someone else, or do I keep trying, attack it?

I decided to keep trying. Basketball at my high school was king—a rich tradition of conference, regional, and state championships. I waited a year, watching games from the stands and feeling jealous and perhaps a bit bitter. But those emotions fueled my determination to work on my game, waiting for next year's tryouts to prove that I deserved to be on that team. I was glad that I had been cut. It made me mad. I'll show them; they cut the wrong kid. Revenge is a powerful motivator, and so is a dream. I had both. Years later, that same revenge was directed at my diabetes, and later at my goal to race the Ironman triathlon. Diabetes would attack the wrong guy.

I wanted to make that basketball team, but I was not broadcasting it; I had quiet, private, almost angry determination. I would repeat that later in life too. I showed up at varsity tryouts the next fall. After three weeks of workouts, drills, and scrimmages, the time came for another list. Why does there always have to be a list?

As I had the year before, I walked into the lobby of the gymnasium, scanned the list of names typed on the sheet of paper titled "J.L. Mann Varsity Basketball Team." I was not on the list. Ugh. I got cut. Again. Just like last year. I felt as though there was another list posted beside that one that read "Those Chumps Who Didn't Make it" . . . with my name at the top. Getting cut the year before was a painful test and lesson, and I didn't really need another lesson. More failure. More disappointment. More humiliation. What do I do now?

Some crossroads in life are more significant than others. Being cut from the high school basketball team two years in a row might not seem that significant, but to a fifteen-year-old boy, then sixteen-year-old boy, it was pretty painful. It would shape my character and teach me how to respond when knocked down. If you have just been diagnosed with diabetes, or with any health condition, or received other bad news, been laid off from your job, divorced, lost a loved one—how do you respond?

The fall of my senior year arrived. Time for varsity basketball tryouts again. I had been cut from the junior varsity team as a sophomore. Cut from the varsity team as a junior. This was my last chance. I had been knocked down once, knocked down twice. Do I get up again?

I showed up at tryouts. I had worked hard all summer—shooting, dribbling, running, lifting weights, working on my fitness. I knew I would not be the most skilled player, but I would definitely be the hardest working. Learn your skills and figure out how to make them work. I hoped the coach would at least recognize my hard work and determination to not quit. But at six-foot three-inches tall, I was a shooting guard, so I still had to be able to make a jump shot and take the ball up the court against a full court press. For three weeks of tryouts, the whole school seemed to be wagering and chatting about who was, and was not, going to make the team. As a seventeen-year-old walking the halls, I felt as though everyone was looking at me with a mix of snickering ("You don't know when to give up, do you, Jay?") or pity ("How are you going to handle getting cut again?")

I stepped into that arena a third time. The list was posted in the same place. Just as I had in the two years before, I walked into the lobby of the gymnasium. Alone. I could not face this moment with others around me. "J.L. Mann Varsity Basketball Team." It was typed just as it had been two years before: thirteen names stacked on top of each other.

I scanned the names. I saw all the ones I expected to see. My heart sank and pounded. Why did I put myself through this? You idiot. Can't you find something a little easier to shoot for? Do they have a senior superlative in the yearbook for "Most Likely to Never Get the Message and Be Too Stupid to Sacrifice Himself Three Years in a Row and Get Cut from the Basketball Team?"

Maybe I could win that one. It was like a drug that I could not stop trying to get, trying out for that team, only I had never experienced the high—only the low, the hangover.

Then I saw it.

My name.

It was on the list.

I made it!

Mark Twain once said, "Twenty years from now you'll be more disappointed by the things you didn't do than by the things you did." I'm so glad I kept trying, refusing to give up. It helped me then, and it helped me six years later when diabetes entered my life.

Six years later, 1991, after graduating from Wake Forest University, I was in my first year of law school at the University of South Carolina. I was twenty-three years old. Life had been pretty good for me since high school. I had had a great time in college, graduating *cum laude*; I had backpacked on trains through Europe for a few months, then had worked for a couple of years in Washington, D.C. on Capitol Hill. But the first year of law school was psychological warfare. I was in class three to four hours a day and studying five to six hours a day. Not much exercise; just going to classes, studying, and if I had time, maybe sleeping for a few hours at night.

Law school was also full of evil professors tormenting me with the equally evil Socratic method. Traditionally, law school professors don't teach or lecture while you sit passively and listen, as some do in college. Law school professors ask you questions in front of seventy-five other students all hiding behind their desks, humiliate you if you have not read the material, or surgically carve up your answer until you are a mumbling pile of goo. Tradition demands that first-year law students be humiliated and humbled in order to see who will quit and drop out. I thought it really was just a way to torment law students.

Most law students are driven and bright, and grades are determined by one final exam at the end of each semester, not by multiple tests throughout the semester. For the first five months of law school, there is a lot of pressure to make good grades in order to get a summer job, which in turn leads to future jobs. But I was determined to get through: Oh, you think you can make me quit? Just watch. I proved that in high school, trying to make the basketball team.

But that's when I got sick. First semester law school was miserable, so I was supposed to feel miserable, right? As fall and winter arrived—cold, dark, wet weather, stressful first-semester final exams in December—I was not exercising much, just reading, studying, and no doubt stressing. In January 1991, I remember feeling as though I had a cold and a sore throat. I felt gradually weaker. As it got worse, I just thought I had the flu. Soon I could not even walk with my book bag (law books are about two inches thick) from my car, across the large parking lot, and up the stairs to the classroom without stopping to rest.

My throat was so sore I would stop at the fast food restaurant across from the law school to get a frosty ice cream or sweet iced tea. Sweet tea in the South is one part tea, five parts sugar. I did not know it then, but I was just "poisoning" myself with sugar.

But I did not have time to be sick. If I missed even one class, much less a whole day, I would fall hopelessly behind, and the professor would target me the next day like a predator drone strike. I was twenty-three, sharing an apartment with my twenty-five-year-old brother, who was also in graduate school at the University of South Carolina. We studied and went to classes and often did not see each other for days. No one was spotting the signs of my body: weight loss, severe thirst, pale skin, dark eyes. But everyone looked pretty bad in the winter of the first year of law school. No one around me knew what diabetes was or what high blood sugar looked like.

During those days of weakness, I simply trudged through the days like a zombie. I remember one person commenting that my breath smelled "fruity," which I know now is a symptom of *ketoacidosis*. *Ketoacidosis* occurs from prolonged high blood glucose (*hyperglycemia*) caused by the lack of insulin. It causes the liver to break down fat and protein for energy, creating excessive acid in the blood. Glucose (sugar) overloads the kidneys and spills into the urine, causing dehydration as the body tries to flush this excessive glucose from the blood stream. In extreme cases, *diabetic ketoacidosisis* is potentially life threatening.

After a few weeks of fighting a losing battle against this "cold," getting weaker and weaker, I finally admitted that I needed to see a doctor. My student health insurance policy required me to first visit the school's infirmary. I had a brief visit with a physician (or perhaps a medical resident, I don't know, I was pretty delirious) with many questions, trying to diagnose my symptoms. He probably asked questions about diabetes and other potential conditions, and I probably denied any knowledge of diabetes because there was no history of it in my family. I didn't even know what it was. It was late in the afternoon. He said they needed a fasting blood test, so I had to return the next morning to give blood. Ugh. A big needle. Okay. I'll be back tomorrow morning.

I spent a miserable night—nauseous and weak, unable to sleep, up every two hours to urinate. The next morning finally came. I remember being so weak that I could not hold my arm up long enough to shave my face. But I followed instructions not to eat breakfast so that I could give a fasting blood test. My throat was very dry and sore, so I drank some cold orange juice with ice. That didn't count, right? I was still fasting. I had not *eaten* anything. I went to the infirmary, struggling to walk from the parking lot, feeling like my head was full of water and going to explode. They told me, "Sorry, you have to come back." That orange juice counted. They needed a fasting blood test. No food, no fruit juice. Come back tomorrow morning.

What followed was the worst day and night of my life. I lay in bed all day. That night I hallucinated and heard voices and sounds, saw colors like trains barreling though my skull spewing psychedelic rainbow colors behind them. I was nauseous, crawling to the bathroom and hanging on the toilet to vomit, then dry heave, unsuccessfully, since I had not felt like eating much that day. I also had to urinate constantly but could hardly sit on the toilet. I staggered back to my bed and lapsed in and out of sleep or consciousness. The next morning my brother found me in the apartment. I barely remember talking to him, but I definitely remember hanging onto his shoulders as he dragged me from his car up the sidewalk to the infirmary, like a teammate carrying an injured player off the field. I collapsed at the infirmary and woke up several hours later in the university hospital's emergency room.

I had tubes in my nose and an intravenous drip in my arm. An endocrinologist was standing over me, but I did not know she was an endocrinologist. She was just a doctor in a white lab coat. I was so weak I could not lift my head.

"Hi Jay. I'm Dr. McFarland."

I blinked, looked at her, trying to figure out where I was and what had happened to me. Had I been in a car accident? Perhaps there was some other minor discussion in which I was too weak to engage. Then she told me.

"Jay, your blood sugar is dangerously high. You have diabetes."

She was a gentle, soft-spoken woman, and no doubt had had this conversation with patients and families before. After contemplating this for a few minutes, I remember asking her three questions:

"What's diabetes?" I had never seen it or even heard of it. There was no history of it in my family. No type 1 or type 2 diabetes in my parents, grandparents, brother, sister, cousins, aunts, or uncles.

She told me about diabetes.

"Am I going to die?" I'm sure tears were in my eyes. I was too weak to hold them back. I was hearing all of this alone. This sounded serious. Something was wrong with my blood. I could go blind, have my foot amputated. I could have kidney failure, go on dialysis. Was she telling me everything? I would have to test my blood every day and take injections with a syringe. Shots every day, multiple times a day. For the rest of my life.

"No," she said, "you're not going to die. At least not today." She paused and looked at me, deep into my eyes. "But your life is going to change."

"Is there a cure?"

"No." She paused. "There's no cure. Not today."

In the days, weeks, and months after that, I adjusted to life with type 1 diabetes. Type 1 is insulin-dependent diabetes. They still called it Juvenile Diabetes in 1991 because that form of diabetes attacks most people as kids, but I suppose I was part of changing that term since it hit me at age twenty-three. It was not the "dark ages" of diabetes, with urine strips to detect sugar or boiling needles for insulin, but in 1991 I did catch the tail end of using pork insulin, and my first blood sugar meter required forty-five seconds. We did not have tools like insulin pumps or convenient insulin pens.

It was a blow to my self-confidence, realizing that my body was not invincible. I had lived twenty-three years of "normal" life—eating, drinking, doing whatever I wanted without worrying about blood sugar, carbohydrates, or the effect of exercise. Now I had a chronic condition with no cure. It required constant daily management, calculating carbohydrates in everything I ate. I was carrying around meters and test strips, hiding syringes and a vial of insulin in my book bag, injecting myself in the bathroom stall like a heroin addict. I was never depressed, but I was shaken.

I continued through law school, suffering only a few bad episodes of low blood sugar (*hypoglycemia*), but I never ended up in the hospital. Fortunately my roommates were able to help me at those times. I loaded up on sugar-free foods and diet drinks in the grocery store. Some of those were humorous mistakes. One day I was excited to find sugar-free chocolate in the grocery store. I loved chocolate. I ate almost the whole bag. After an unusual number of trips to the bathroom that day, I read the label on the bag: "Sweetened with sorbitol. Excessive consumption may have a laxative effect." Yes, indeed, it may.

After graduation, I began working as a young lawyer for a big law firm in South Carolina with about fifty lawyers. I kept my diabetes private, except for those who needed to know. I did not want others to view me as sick. I was single, living alone, working long hours in the salt mine of a large law firm. It was the mid 1990s, and I was using the old Regular and NPH insulins, so the timing of when insulin would peak was often a "W-A-G"—a *wild-ass guess*. After injecting Regular insulin, I had to wait thirty minutes to eat. Would the NPH insulin peak in three hours or four hours today? It was as if the "diabetes guy" would follow me around all day, hiding in the shadows and crowd, waiting for the moment when I least expected it, then suddenly jumping out of nowhere and hitting me in the face with the *hypoglycemia* boxing glove. BAM!! Take that!!. . . leaving me dazed, wobbly, and stumbling . . . then he'd disappear in the crowd and not appear again for days.

I tried to have carbohydrate drinks and food handy to fend off low blood sugar reactions and checked my blood sugar as often as possible, but I was not always successful. I remember getting ready for work early one morning in my apartment, thinking it was a normal morning, and waking up several hours later on the floor, sweating in my dress shirt and pants. I don't know what I did or did not do to cause that low blood sugar reaction that morning, but somehow that "diabetes guy" got into my apartment and clocked me so hard in the face, in my kitchen, that it knocked me out. Fortunately I awoke and was able to get myself some glucose and recover. But it scared the crap out of me. My endocrinologist later told me that it was not a good idea for me to live alone or sleep alone. I asked if he could write me a prescription for that. As a single guy in my twenties, I thought that would be a pretty good pick-up line: "Hey, my doctor says I'm not supposed to sleep alone. See, I have a doctor's note."

I was doing everything I could to follow the best blood sugar management regimen available in the mid 1990s. I was trying to live my life as if I did not have diabetes. But I was not living in denial; I was living in determination. Determination to prove that diabetes would not stop me from doing anything. I respected my diabetes, but I would not surrender to it. I exercised, ran a little, lifted weights, but I did not swim, bike, or run competitively. I didn't even own a bike or have a membership at a pool.

After a few years of living with this disease, I wanted to prove that I was stronger than my diabetes. I needed a challenge, something hard. Everyone needs goals, but not just any goals: goals with failure potential. Goals that you might not achieve the first time, or maybe the second time, but that are so much more satisfying when you do achieve them. I learned that trying out for the basketball team in high school. If you have never failed, you are setting your goals too low, and you are not as successful as you could be. Failure is good. Don't be afraid to fail. In fact, embrace failure. Learn from it. Now you have something to shoot for.

My first goal with failure potential with diabetes happened in 1999. I got a flyer in my mailbox about running a marathon to raise money for the American Diabetes Association (ADA). I had never run a marathon in my life. If I raised enough money, they'd send me to Hawaii to run this marathon. It seemed like a pretty good deal—raise money for a diabetes charity, take on the challenge of running a marathon, and run it in a place where I wanted to be when I was finished. It also gave me comfort to run a marathon with a coach who gave me workouts. I hoped that I would have people around who understood diabetes— even though I was the only one with diabetes doing the marathon from my area.

I trained for months and ran the marathon in June. It was 26.2 miles of the most difficult, painful, miserable . . . wonderful miles of my life. It was the hardest thing I had ever done, and I loved every excruciating minute of it. I crossed that finish line, and it was about nine hundred degrees in Hawaii. Lying on the ground in the shade at that finish line while others were finishing, I felt miserable, exhausted, a bit nauseous, completely dehydrated . . . and very proud of myself. I had just run a marathon with type 1 diabetes. I had proven that diabetes would not stop me from doing one of the most difficult things in life— run a marathon. But I was exhausted. Stick a fork in me; I was done.

Then this guy sitting next to me leaned over. "You know, this is where they run the Ironman Triathlon. Those guys swim two and a half miles out there in the Pacific Ocean. Then they bike 112 miles up to Hawaii and back . . . and *then* they run this marathon."

I rolled my head over to that guy. And I threw up on him. What kind of freak of fitness can do that?! Swim two and a half miles, bike 112 miles, and then run this marathon? And who could do that with type 1 diabetes?

But right then I had another goal: a goal with a lot more failure potential then just running a marathon. I was going to do the Ironman triathlon. I was going to do it with type 1 diabetes. For two years I worked for that goal. I ran two other marathons in Rome, Italy and Kona, Hawaii raising money for the ADA. I borrowed a fifteen-year-old road bike from one of my co-workers and rode seventy-five miles in the ADA's *Ride to Cure* charity ride. I bought my own road bike and started riding a lot. I joined a pool and started swimming. The first few times, I could barely swim two lengths of the pool without stopping to rest. I knew how to swim for fun but not for speed or distance. My first triathlon was an Olympic-distance race, just a 1,500-meter swim, 24-mile bike, and a 10k run, and I trained for that like I was in the Olympics. I was nervous but also focused and obsessed to some day race an Ironman triathlon.

While I was learning to swim, bike, and run like a triathlete, and learning the equipment for the sport—swim goggles, wetsuit, bike, cycling shoes and apparel, helmet, running shoes and apparel—I also had a lot to learn about sport nutrition: sport drinks, gels, and bars. I was also learning to balance my blood sugar, insulin dosing, and diabetes equipment of blood sugar meters, strips, and insulin pump for workouts and the race. I had to learn about pre-workout fueling to keep my blood sugar up during workouts, and post-workout fueling to keep my blood sugar from crashing after long workouts and during the night. It was a lot of trial and error, experimenting with high-carbohydrate meals one hour before long bike rides or runs in the morning—oatmeal was a favorite— and large pasta meals for dinner after several hours on the bike or running.

Sometimes I learned this lesson the hard way in my first year of training. One amateur bike race on July 4th was seventy miles in the mountains of western North Carolina near my home in upstate South Carolina. After seventy miles of very hot, very hard cycling, I drove the one-hour return trip home, stopping to pick up a salad with chicken and some bread. Not a lot of carbohydrates in that meal. I was supposed to meet some friends later that evening, about three hours away, at the beach. I ate the meal, *bolused* the insulin, and packed at home, but I was so exhausted that I lay down on my sofa for what I thought would be a quick nap and dropped into a dangerously low *hypoglycemic* state. I essentially lost consciousness, woke up several hours later, covered in sweat, unable to stand or communicate. Somehow I managed to have a few flashes of coherent thought to realize that I was in *hypoglycemic shock*. I was jerking and jumping, hands and fingers twitching. I knocked the phone off the table nearby but could not punch the buttons or even know what to do with it if I could have remembered what numbers to punch, including 911. I rolled onto the floor for about thirty minutes (I assume), struggled to crawl and drag myself about twenty feet to my kitchen, and collapsed in the pantry beneath a shelf where I kept some Sprite® sodas. I managed to reach up and grab a six-pack of cans and pulled them down crashing on my chest, my hands jerking and trembling. Fingers, legs, and arms don't work in *severe hypoglycemia*. Your glucose-deprived brain cannot control your muscles or direct your body to perform the most simple of tasks.

I don't know how long it took me to pry open one of those cans of Sprite® as I lay on the floor, twitching and fumbling, but eventually I got one to my mouth and poured it on my face, sucking some in. As I lay there, I slowly, gradually, regained some consciousness. I was covered in sweat and Sprite®, and the path from my sofa to the kitchen was wrecked because I had dragged myself across the carpet and between furniture from one room to the next. That was a scary, valuable lesson. After that, I ate large carbohydrate meals of pasta and lowered my insulin dosage after long, hard workouts and races.

After two years of training, racing marathons, doing bike training rides and laps in the pool, and completing several Olympic-distance and Half Ironman triathlons, I crossed the finish line of my very first Ironman triathlon in 2002. I did it on a road bike with clip-on aero bars rather than on an official triathlon-racing bike. I worked very hard to maintain my blood sugar throughout the 140.6-mile race. After swimming 2.4 miles, then cycling 112 miles, the marathon was a 26.2-mile suffer fest, but it was the same for every athlete in the Ironman. I wore an insulin pump with a tube and my infusion set stuck in my upper buttocks. I took the pump off for the swim, then reattached it for the 112-mile bike ride and the marathon, wearing it clipped to the belt around my waist with the tube pumping insulin dangling and wrapped around my waist into my triathlon shorts at my butt.

That first Ironman was difficult, but I loved every mile of it. I crossed that finish line after 140.6 miles of swimming, cycling, and running in just over eleven hours. They will let athletes stay out on the course for seventeen hours, so I did okay for my very first one. I cried at the finish line—tears of joy and satisfaction. I was an Ironman. An Ironman with diabetes. Maybe others in the race did not know how hard it was to do it trying to manage my blood sugar, but I did.

At the finisher's banquet the next day, I was very proud of myself. I wanted to find that guy I had puked on at the finish line of my first marathon two years before in Hawaii when he told me about the Ironman, and say "How do you like me now?"

At that Ironman finisher's banquet, they started calling out the times of the top finishers in the race, athletes from all over the world: Australia, Germany, Spain, Czech Republic. Those guys had done the race two hours faster than I had. Two hours! They were not even in the same race that I was in. They had enough time to cross the finish line, get a shower, go to a movie, drop by Starbucks and return a few emails, then come back and watch my sorry sack of flesh come rolling and stumbling across the finish line.

I was in awe. Those guys were super human: amazing physical specimens, strong and fast, and so fit. They were on their national teams, some on the Team USA national team for long distance triathlon. I about lost a lung and puked a kidney to do it in the time that I did, and those guys did it TWO HOURS faster than I did?

But right then I had another goal, a goal with a lot more failure potential than running a marathon or completing an Ironman. I was going to cut two hours off my time. I was going to qualify for the U.S. National team. I was going to compete with the best Ironman triathletes in the world, and I was going to do it with type 1 diabetes.

For two years I worked for that goal. But to be one of the best, I knew that I had to change the way I had been training and get better equipment. I got a triathlon coach. I bought a time-trial triathlon-racing bike. I started training with elite road cyclists, racing every week with some of the best cyclists in the area, pushing me harder and faster. I took swim technique lessons and changed my swimming technique. I also changed my running technique, doing track workouts, speed work and interval training, and long-distance run training.

You have heard that the definition of insanity is doing the same thing every day and expecting a different result. After that first Ironman, I knew I had to change things to compete with the best triathletes. Unfortunately, many people with diabetes are guilty of doing the same thing over and over and wondering why their blood sugar and hemoglobin A1c readings do not improve. You have to exercise, change to a healthier diet, consult with your doctor and healthcare team about new insulin and delivery systems—such as an insulin pen or an insulin pump—check your blood sugar more frequently and with faster blood sugar meters, or perhaps use a continuous glucose monitor.

I began training fifteen to eighteen hours a week, workouts twice a day during the week, and long workouts of five or six hours on the weekends. I was also working full time, fifty hours a week as a lawyer, so my life was busy with work and training. But you always have time for the things that are important to you. Racing the Ironman was important to me, and of course I was not getting paid to race or to speak at that point, so I had to keep my day job.

On a sample training week, for example, on a Monday, I swam early in the morning for an hour and a half, then ran six or seven miles at lunch or after work when others in my life might be eating lunch or going to happy hour. The next day I did speed work on the track of 400-meter, 800-meter, and 1000-meter intervals, high intense sprint workouts to increase leg turnover, with my heart rate so high I would almost collapse. Then I cycled that evening forty or fifty miles with local elite cyclists at 25 to 30 mph. Wednesdays it was back in the pool at 5:30 a.m. and another run workout later that day. Thursday, I might have done bike-run duathlon workouts: cycle fourteen miles, run two miles, cycle seven miles, run one mile, cycle seven miles, and run two miles to train my body to run off the bike. Fridays were easy days of just a swim workout to prepare for the weekend. Saturdays were long cycling workouts of 80 to 100 miles, then immediate runs of five or six miles. Sundays were long runs of fifteen to twenty miles in the morning, then easy cycling of twenty miles that evening to relax and recover and flush the lactic acid and toxins from my system before starting all over again on Monday. I was very careful to plan my pre- and post-workout nutrition to fuel the workout and maintain my blood sugar and to carry sport bars, gels, sport drinks, and a blood sugar meter with me on long workouts.

During all those hours of training, I was earning my Ironman finish line, and usually no one saw me doing it. Ironman training was often a lonely road: early in the morning, late at night, and on weekends. With a few exceptions (training with some training partners), no one was watching me in the pool, on long cycling workouts, or while running. Once I got married and had my first child, I began swimming before sunrise and doing indoor cycling workouts on my indoor trainer in the basement at 10 p.m. while everyone else was asleep. Work-life balance requires one to prioritize for work and family while striving for another goal.

You don't earn your finish line on race day; you earn it every day when no one is watching you. With thousands of people watching me on race day, I knew I had earned that Ironman finish line by training in the heat and cold, rain and darkness, when no one was watching me. That gave me confidence. I deserved that finish line.

It is the same with diabetes and success in life. You earn your health with the decisions you make every day when no one is watching you. Exercising rather than sitting on the couch when it is cold and rainy in the winter or hot in the summer, eating healthy rather than junk fast food, checking your blood sugar and taking your insulin. That regimen will earn your healthy A1c blood test reading that your doctor sees, but your doctor and healthcare team and family do not see you every day earning that healthy reading. In school, business, athletics, and your health, you earn your promotion, your diploma, your finish line with the decisions you make and things you do when no one is watching you.

Over the next two years of racing Ironman triathlons and shorter triathlons, I was improving my fitness and results in races but still struggling with managing my blood sugar during the Ironman distance. I made mistakes and learned lessons. In my second Ironman triathlon in Lake Placid, New York, I was having a great race on the bike. It was only my second Ironman, but I felt as though I was no longer a rookie and had raced several Half Ironman distance races well. I completed the 2.4-mile swim and was about eighty miles into the bike at the base of a mountain before the thirty miles back into the mountainous village of Lake Placid. With thirty miles to go, I was feeling good and having a great race. I did not want to carry the extra weight of my bottles with carbohydrate sport drink on my bike up the mountain, so I dumped them at the base of a climb with thirty miles to go.

Big mistake! A few miles into that climb, I started to suffer and slow. It was eighty-five miles into the bike race, and I was climbing a mountain, so I expected to slow down, but guys were beginning to catch me, and I could not keep pace with those in front of me. My blood sugar had dropped, but I had dumped my carbohydrate sport drink several miles earlier. The next twenty miles I suffered to turn over the pedals and drag my body up White Face Mountain, losing strength and time, realizing my mistake and cursing myself. All of my strength was gone, even though I was fit and in great physical shape. That was the most frustrating thing for me with diabetes. I may be one of the strongest, fittest, fastest guys in the race, but my blood sugar can destroy all of that and reduce me to weakness, barely able to run or bike. An engine out of gas.

I finally made it into the bike-to-run transition, dismounted my bike, and wobbled into the transition tent. Everyone wobbles after swimming 2.4 miles and biking 112 miles, but I was dealing with low blood sugar. I did a quick check with my blood sugar meter in my transition bag. 42 mg/dL! Ugh. I was weak and exhausted but coherent and not in danger. I had not *bolused* any insulin during the race, so I was not in danger of crashing. It had just been a slow downward blood sugar slide. I sipped for a few minutes on the high carbohydrate drink in my transition bag, then trotted slowly out of the transition tent, sipping on that bottle, and started running (jogging) the 26.2-mile marathon. I lost a lot of time in the last thirty miles of the bike, sitting in transition, and jogging slowly in the early miles of the marathon while waiting for my blood sugar to come up. I learned a valuable lesson.

In the Ironman, I never forget that I have diabetes. But I do forget that the other athletes don't have diabetes. Diabetes is just one more thing in the long list of things that I have to keep up with during the race. But the other athletes are no doubt dealing with their own difficulties as well, some even greater than mine, emotional and physical challenges. I am not a victim, and I do not feel sorry for myself.

My diabetes is a ball and chain attached to my ankle that goes with me every step of my life. But it better be able to swim because I am going to drown it pulling it 2.4 miles in the ocean. And it better have thick skin because I'm going to rip every bit of its flesh off its body dragging it on the asphalt at 22 mph for 112 miles on the bike. It better have strong bones because I'm going to break every bone in its body slamming it on the ground behind me running the 26.2-mile marathon. I will use every muscle, fiber, cell, calorie, and follicle in my body to get to that finish line and collapse in the arms of the race officials. But I always have just enough strength to turn around at the finish line and step on the neck of my diabetes chained to my ankle and say "you are messing with the wrong guy!"

Although the Ironman is so physically demanding, ironically it is the smartest athlete who wins. It is the same with diabetes. You have to be smart and prepared to prevent blood sugar fluctuations and to react when it happens. In the Ironman, you must be fit and strong, but you must also pace yourself and manage your nutrition. Over the course of one Ironman race, I will burn approximately 12,000 calories. I will consume only about 3,000 calories, so I have to metabolize the fat stores in my body for fuel by going as fast as I can with my heart rate down below my anaerobic threshold. I need to consume between sixty and eighty grams of carbohydrate every hour of the race from sport drinks, gels, bars, and other nutrition at the race aid stations. Any less than sixty grams, and I will get low blood sugar and become weak, feeble and shaky; more than eighty grams, and I will run the risk of high blood sugar, nausea, bloating, the need to urinate, and dehydration later in the race. I will drink two to two and one-half gallons of liquid during the race to stay hydrated in the 85°F to 90°F heat for hot-weather races in Florida, Australia, Hawaii, and the Virgin Islands. All of this attention to detail is similar to living life with diabetes. You have to be smart, be prepared, adapt, and react.

After two years of racing and seven Ironman triathlons, I still had not reached my goal to cut two hours off my time and be at the front of the race with the best in the world. In 2004, I was in the seventh Ironman race of my career. I was beginning to wonder if diabetes would prevent me from being one of the best. I had had a miserable year that year, racing Ironman Coeur d'Alene, Idaho in June and failing to finish because I got so dehydrated that I collapsed at mile eighteen of the marathon, 132 miles into the race. My dehydration had been caused by high blood sugar four hours earlier on the bike, causing my body to try to flush out all of the excess glucose in my blood by urinating while trying to hydrate to race the Ironman triathlon. It was a hydration battle that I lost.

The week after Ironman Coeur d'Alene, I flew to Sweden and raced the ITU Long Distance Triathlon World Championship with the U.S. National team: two long distance triathlons in six days on two different continents of the globe. Not the ideal schedule, but I had qualified for Team USA earlier in the year and already had Idaho on my schedule. I was excited that I seemed to be on my way to racing with the best, but I still had not put together a great race to finish with the best. The U.S. team doctors and physiotherapists worked on my body that week in Sweden, helping me recover from my disastrous race in Idaho. I raced the ITU World Championship for Team USA and did okay, but I finished in the middle of the pack, disappointed that I was fitter and faster than my result showed. Just like Ironman Idaho, my blood sugar got too high again during the bike, then dropped too low on the run; dehydration was also a problem again. Proper nutrition was difficult for me to figure out.

Back in the United States, I raced Ironman Wisconsin six weeks later, and had a good swim and a good bike, but I got nauseous early in the marathon. I threw up at mile three of the marathon, and several more times, until I finally was reduced to walking the last eighteen miles of that marathon. I could have walked off the course at any point and disappeared into the crowd, but I was determined to walk every step of that marathon even though I could not run. I spent eighteen miles questioning whether I had the ability to race with the best in the world. Would diabetes stop me from doing it? What could I do differently? For how many more races would I do this?

My fourth Ironman race of that year was in November in Florida. Four Ironman triathlons in one year was a lot of racing, but my fitness and race strength were on target. However, I was struggling to figure out the proper nutrition to keep my blood sugar stable during the race. In the weeks leading up to that race, I had changed my nutrition plan, tried different things in training, and had success in shorter Half Ironman distance races. It was now or never. Could I make it work in this, my seventh Ironman race of my career, to finally race with the leaders, the best in the world?

Ironically, this race in Florida was also the site of my very first Ironman race two years before. If I was going to cut two hours off my time, this was the race in which to do it, on the same course where I had started as a rookie two years prior. I needed to swim 2.4 miles in one hour, bike 112 miles in under five hours, and then run the marathon under three and one-half hours. I also could not waste time in transition; I needed fast blood sugar checks and no mechanical problems. I had a great swim and bike and started the marathon at about 1 p.m. in 85°F heat; everything was going right. I was up front with the leaders. I felt strong on the early portions of the marathon. My blood sugar was staying stable, and I was eating gels and bars and drinking sport drinks and water on schedule, staying hydrated.

After racing 134 miles, I was at mile twenty of that marathon, with only six miles left to run. I was hurting pretty bad, but everybody hurts at that point of the race. At that point, two athletes passed me, one from Germany and one from the United States. They were good marathon runners who had caught me after twenty miles of that marathon after I had got ahead of them on the bike. I started running behind them for several miles, struggling to hold their pace. At mile 137 of the race I had only three more miles to go, and I was dying. The pain was indescribable. Searing muscle pain in my legs from 137 miles of racing, lactic acid burning the muscles with a deep piercing pain in my quads like someone was jamming a fork into my leg with each step. Struggling to breathe like someone was tightening a belt around my chest and pouring battery acid down my throat.

The crowd lining the route of the last three miles of the Ironman will cheer, trying to lift you up and carry you to the finish. They know that each runner is hurting, struggling, fighting the pain and doubt and longing for that finish line. That crowd had not seen me earning my finish line all of those days that I had been training alone, miles and miles of cycling and running and laps in the pool. That crowd had not seen me in that hospital bed in 1991, or when low blood sugar made it hard to even think, much less exercise, and high blood sugar made me sick.

I deserved that finish line. I was on pace to cut two hours off my first Ironman time and to finish with the best in the world. But now I was struggling. My blood sugar had dropped *below* 80 mg/dL at that point (I know only because I checked it after the race). I could lose thirty minutes, even an hour, if I had to slow or stop the last three miles of the race. I had come so far, raced for seven Ironman triathlons, three bad Ironmans that year, 137 miles of racing that day, and it all came down to those last three miles. I barely hung on. I didn't think I could keep going. My dream was slipping through my fingers.

And then during that race, when I was struggling just to keep going, out of the crowd, I saw my coach. He shouted one thing to me as I went by.

"How bad do you want it?"

He could have shouted some training tip, or something about my technique, but he knew that did not matter at that point. All that mattered was how bad I wanted it.

I wanted it for the 10,000 times I had stuck myself with a syringe, injected insulin three, four, or five times a day in the thirteen years since I had been diagnosed. I wanted it for the 50,000 times I had pricked my finger, dropping blood on a glucose meter, testing my blood sugar six, seven, sometimes eight times a day. I wanted it for all the kids with diabetes whom I had heard from in my racing and who had written me letters and emails having seen me in magazines, and the adults with diabetes, all wondering if they or their kids could overcome diabetes.

But I really wanted it, for that one moment in time, to be more than I thought I could be that day in the emergency room in 1991 when that doctor told me I had diabetes and that my life was going to change. She was right. My life had changed. Changed for the better.

A fire erupted in me, and I raced the last three miles of that Ironman. I got to the last 150 meters of that finishing chute with tears in my eyes. I was slapping the hands of the spectators as I went by, soaking up the music, the crowd, and the noise. I crossed the finish line in 9 hours, 47 minutes, and 14 seconds—almost two hours faster than I had in the same race just two years before. I was now up there with the best triathletes in the world.

I have raced many triathlons since that day: fourteen Ironmans, over twenty Half Ironmans, and dozens of Olympic-distance and sprint triathlons. I raced for three years on the U.S. National Team USA at the ITU Long Distance Triathlon World Championships in Denmark, Sweden, and Australia. I've raced many marathons by themselves, including three times at the Boston Marathon. I have raced a lot of bike races, including the Race Across America with my friends, Phil Southerland and Joe Eldridge, in the early days of Team Type 1, racing 3,130 miles across the United States on our bikes in 5 days and 16 hours.

Diabetes has been my motivation to race, to prove that I could overcome it, that I am stronger than it is.

Make diabetes the best thing that ever happened to you. I would not be racing the Ironman if I did not have diabetes. Use it as motivation to eat healthy, exercise, prove that you can manage it. Set goals and do not be afraid to fail; be smart and keep trying. Earn your finish line with hard work, discipline, dedication, and the decisions you make when no one is watching you.

I am now a motivational speaker, running my business called Finish Line Vision. (For further information, please see the website at the conclusion of this chapter.) I speak to companies and organizations all over the world about achieving goals in life and business. Achieving finish lines. Overcoming obstacles. Keeping a healthy lifestyle and work-life balance. I am also the author of my motivational book, *Finish Line Vision*.

None of this would have happened if I had not been diagnosed with diabetes. That doctor was right: my life was going to change, and I am glad that it did.

Keep going. You will get to your finish line.

www.finishlinevision.com

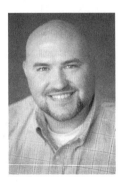

CHAPTER 10   *by Scott Johnson*

Your Strength is Showing Again...

I woke up fighting through a cloud of confusion. I opened my eyes to find two strangers standing next to me, one on each side. The guy on my right held an intravenous bag above his head. I followed the attached line with my eyes to find the other end of the line poking into my arm. The guy on the left was asking questions. "Do you know what year it is?" and "What is your name?"

And then it all made sense. It was the middle of the night on Thursday, February 24, 2000, and I was recovering from the first low blood sugar seizure in over fifteen years. I knew exactly why it happened, and I felt really stupid.

I had been playing basketball early in the evening when my insulin pump infusion set came out. Thinking that I'd be okay to finish playing, I had just let it go for a while. I probably would have been just fine, but my blood sugar was probably running high, and I was possibly dehydrated before starting. By the third or fourth game, my calf muscles were cramping, and I had no energy.

Sure enough, testing my blood sugar after I finished playing showed that I was near 400 mg/dL. I took some insulin through a syringe, but after about an hour, the level had not gone down at all. In fact, now my blood sugar was *over* 500 mg/dL. Back home, I took some more insulin through a syringe, put in a new infusion set for my pump, and took a bit more insulin for good measure.

Without thinking much about it, I had just performed a *rage serial bolus.* A *rage bolus* means dialing up a large amount of insulin, usually significantly more than what is needed, to bring down a stubborn high blood sugar. *Serial bolusing* means taking *bolus* upon *bolus,* trying to bring down a stubborn high blood sugar. Usually, either one of these tactics alone is enough to get you in trouble. I combined them both. And I knew better.

But there I went, wildly stacking large doses of insulin on top of each other, trying to avoid trouble with high blood sugars. Then I made the ultimate mistake.

I went to bed.

The EMTs asked my wife to bring me a peanut butter and jelly sandwich, and they stayed while I ate it.

As they were leaving, my wife's parents showed up; they lived just down the street. A few minutes later, my parents arrived; they lived on the other side of the city. Did I mention it was the middle of the night? I felt very guilty for bothering all of my parents. I had done this to myself, and it was my fault that everyone was awake and at my house worried about me. I was upset with myself for letting my diabetes spill out into their lives in such an inconvenient way.

My wife wouldn't talk about it for a long time. When she finally did, I understood why she hadn't wanted to talk about it. I was seizing and convulsing, which alone must have been terrifying. Then, while she was on the phone with 911, I just stopped. With the phone in one hand, and our month-old son in the other, she thought she had just witnessed her husband die.

No wonder she called our parents. Poor thing.

I felt so guilty. I felt ashamed for not being able to keep the chaos of diabetes inside. I had let my diabetes strike a fear into my wife that I pray she will never experience again.

Four days later, still wrestling with the emotional fallout, I started writing about my life with diabetes. That was over twelve years ago. As I look back on it now, I feel much more forgiving of myself. I see all sorts of mistakes that I made that evening, but I also recognize that, at the time, I was trying my best to avoid *ketoacidosis*. I was maybe a little too successful in that.

My pancreas is broken. That is to blame, not I. As I try my best to manually replicate the work of a divinely designed internal organ, there are sure to be many more mistakes and lessons; all in all, though, I'm doing a pretty good job.

Diagnosis

I was diagnosed with type 1 diabetes in April of 1980. I was five years old—fifteen days after my fifth birthday. I was so young. It's no surprise that I can't remember much about my hospital stay, my first shot, or anything else from back then. But I do have little memories from here and there as I was growing up.

I remember wanting to do my own shots at an early age. I worried that other people would hit something if I let them do it—as if there are all sorts of important and painful organs and stuff just below the skin.

I remember my mom having arguments on the telephone with the insurance company and the pharmacy. Home blood glucose testing was available in the early 1980s, but like anything new, insurance companies didn't want to pay for it.

I remember having to wake up early, even on weekends, to take my shot and have breakfast. Even though it took only a few minutes to test my blood sugar, take my shot, then slam down a glass of milk with chocolate Carnation® Instant Breakfast mix, I remember it being a pain in the butt. What kid wants to think about an alarm clock on the weekends?

I remember filling up used gallon milk containers with my old syringes. It was an "at-home" sharps system that my mom, a nurse, would take to her hospital once it was filled.

I remember carrying two fruit roll-ups in my back pocket in case my blood sugar went low. They would be flattened beyond recognition by the time I finished even a single day of school.

I remember waking up with the most incredible headaches after a few childhood seizures. They always happened at night, and my parents were able to pull me through them using the *glucagon* emergency kits.

I remember passing out in the lunch line in 7th or 8th grade. I had a carton of chocolate milk in my hand but was worried that I'd get in trouble if I didn't pay for it first. I kept wishing the line would hurry up so I could drink my milk, then out I went.

I remember bits and pieces of diabetes camp, called "Camp Needlepoint." I went for about three years in a row and got miserably sick each and every time. It was because of peanut butter. That was during the Exchange System diet, which we never really followed closely at home. I didn't eat much protein, and I disliked meat. But at camp, if I didn't eat my meat, I had to replace the meat with some other protein source. At nearly every meal, I would approach the nutrition counter to trade my meat for a Dixie® cup full of creamy peanut butter. After a few days of forcing all of this peanut butter into my system, I'd spend the next twelve hours in the infirmary puking my guts out. I remember telling the nurse I had to puke, and she gave me this cute little kidney-shaped container to puke in. It was barely big enough to spit in. I told her she'd better get an ice cream bucket or something unless she wanted to be cleaning up an even bigger mess.

I remember spending the entire day at local parks playing basketball as a teenager. I can't believe that I don't remember it being a big deal. Today, it takes so much planning and preparation just to exercise for a short while. How on earth did I manage to spend the whole day at the park without packing a suitcase full of food?

I remember diabetes at school not being much of a big deal either (other than the one time I mentioned above). We didn't have *basal/bolus* therapy like we do now, so I would have taken a single shot in the morning and maybe one in the evening. I'm sure my parents talked to people at the school and knew the nurses pretty well, but from my perspective, there wasn't much to it. A lot can be said for the ignorant resilience of children, right? I also credit the relentless efforts of my mom and dad. They worked hard to keep me from feeling different because of diabetes.

One of the most important lessons that I remember from growing up with diabetes was something my mom taught me. She told me to never use diabetes as an excuse to not do something because, as soon as I did, other people would too, but they'd do so without my permission.

Writing and Growing

As I started writing about my life with diabetes, many things started bubbling to the surface. Being diagnosed at such a young age, I couldn't possibly understand what it meant, nor could I deal with all of the emotions and grief that a chronic diagnosis brings. Once again, the ignorant resilience of childhood amazes me.

Many of the feelings that were surfacing felt vague and unclear, yet extremely important and powerful. They felt like something I needed to work through, but they also frightened me a bit. Writing about them helped me deal with that fear. The exercise of having to assign words and phrases to these feelings continues to be very therapeutic for me.

As I continued to grow and mature, I found that I often had to deal with new and uncharted emotions and feelings around my life with diabetes. I don't think acceptance is a one-time thing; rather, as you face new challenges with diabetes, you have to cope with them and travel again through the grief process. I visit the acceptance phase on a pretty regular cycle, and I am learning that, just because I was there once, doesn't mean I'm there for good.

The connections I've found through writing and sharing online have been incredibly positive and inspiring and I know that, without them, I wouldn't be doing as well as I am today. If you had searched for information ten years ago, what would you have found? The results of your search would have been mostly medical information that described all of the complications and ugly statistics of diabetes. That is not the case anymore. Today, your search will yield countless stories of people living well with diabetes! There are stories of people raising families, having fulfilling careers, and sharing positive and encouraging examples of their lives with diabetes.

We are actively changing what people find when they look for diabetes information, and there are so many of us sharing that nobody can keep up anymore. How awesome is that? We are also normalizing diabetes: we are sharing the whole story of diabetes, not just the good moments. We are sharing the successes, the struggles, and everything in-between. Doing that is extremely important.

Growing up, I had this picture of diabetes perfection in my mind. Every time I had a high or a low, or my A1c result came back high, I felt like a failure. I felt that I wasn't trying hard enough, or that I didn't have the willpower to do what needed to be done. I felt that I was the only person living with diabetes who just couldn't get my act together.

But you know what? That is normal. The struggle is normal. There are more of us struggling to figure out the recipe for success than there are those who are perfect! That's because NOBODY is perfect! How different would your life with diabetes be if you were told, right from the start, how difficult diabetes is to manage? Lord knows, I would have been so much kinder and more forgiving of myself. Instead, I'm still working to shake the burden of guilt that I've built up over the years.

Diabetes is a difficult thing to manage. As long as we wake up each day and try our best, always looking for some new information or strategies to help us do better, we are succeeding.

What is Success?

What exactly is "success" when it comes to diabetes?

A few years ago, my dad helped me track down my health records from when I was growing up. In 1988, which would have put me at age thirteen, I had an A1c of 17.9%. That meant that my average blood sugar was over 500 mg/dL. For three months. This was not right after diagnosis; it was after nearly eight years of diabetes experience. I don't remember what was going through my head, but it couldn't have been pretty.

I have memories of failure, or of not trying hard enough, but when I read the clinicians notes in my records, I don't see the same picture. The picture in my records showed a kid who was trying hard but wrestling with all that diabetes is. I saw a young person who was talking openly about the challenges and working with the healthcare team to come up with different approaches. Some of those approaches worked, and others didn't, and there was no blame. We took a step back and tried something different.

Ever since that time, there has been a slow and steady improvement in my A1c, and I hope that trend continues for the rest of my life. Although the closer I get to a healthy target A1c, the harder it is to stay there and it becomes much harder to improve.

With that in mind, I define success with diabetes as simply never giving up. Every day I wake up (success!) and do my best (success!) to find the balance between satisfactory diabetes management (success!) and great quality of life (success!).

I recognize that I am always reaching for that balance, because it isn't something that stands still. That line moves and changes as much as my blood sugars do, and the fact that I quietly display my strength by constantly striving for better is one of the loudest proclamations of success that I can think of.

www.scottsdiabetes.com

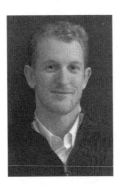

CHAPTER 11   *by Charlie Kimball*

Living in the Fast Lane with Diabetes

There are days in a man's life that change everything. For some, it could be graduating college and getting that first job offer. Maybe it's getting married, or having children. For me, it was my type 1 diabetes diagnosis date: October 16th, 2007. But to really tell my story, you have to go back even further.

A Passion for Speed

As the son of a mechanical engineer who designed race cars for a living, I literally grew up at race tracks. His job took us around the world and frequently took him away from our family on race weekends. Even at a young age, cars always fascinated me, and my passion for racing quickly became apparent to my family. So I started racing go-karts at the age of nine in Southern California. It started as more of a hobby and an opportunity to spend quality time with Dad, but I knew right away that I felt most at home behind the wheel of a car.

Within the next few years I began showing speed and potential on the track, winning more and more go-karting championships—seven national karting championships total. By the time I could get my driver's license, it was evident that racing had become an important part of my life, more than just a weekend hobby. Each trophy fueled my passion for driving and pushed me to get better. For my sixteenth birthday, my parents threw me a surprise party... lots of friends, decorations, cake, the whole deal. The last present I opened was a big box from my mom and dad. I pulled out a white fire suit and then a Nomex® flame resistant undershirt. I was a little confused at first—we didn't need to wear fire suits in karting. Finally, Mom and Dad couldn't hold it in any longer. My big surprise was a two-day test in a Formula Ford, my first open-wheel race car! This was a big step for me. Open-wheel cars are more technologically sophisticated—and much faster—than go-karts. When you look at an open-wheel car you'll see how it gets its name, from the wheels placed outside the car's body, which is different from street cars, stock cars and sports cars. My dad still talks about being able to see my smile through the visor of my helmet after that first lap in the Formula Ford car... I was definitely hooked.

After high school graduation, my next step was largely unknown. I had been accepted into Stanford University's engineering program. It was a tough decision, but I decided to defer my entry. The entire time I was racing go-karts, my mom's main rule was "B's don't race." I had worked hard all through school, and I would have enjoyed following in my father's footsteps, but I knew deep down that I still had more to do behind the wheel of a race car.

At the time, the open-wheel development system was somewhat unsettled in the United States. It was too early for me to join the Atlantic Series, but I was too advanced to continue go-karting. So when an opportunity became available to race an open-wheel car in Europe, I jumped on it.

The Diagnosis

I made some pretty good strides in Europe's racing world, capturing two wins and five pole positions in my first year overseas in British Formula Ford. In 2005, I became the first American in eleven years to win a British Formula 3 race. That year, I won five races and six poles, and I set two track records on the way to finishing second in the championship. I quickly began moving up the ladder in Europe. The following year, I became the first American to win a race in the Formula 3 Euroseries.

There were still a lot of unknowns. I was basically living by myself in a foreign country with lots of firsts—paying bills, doing my own laundry and making my own meals. Driving the race car was the easy part; every other aspect was an adjustment. Little did I know then that I would soon be making even more life alterations.

By 2007, I was settling into the World Series by Renault, a new field of competition for me. The cars were pretty quick—I think I hit 190 mph in the first race—but I was learning and getting better every weekend. After racing in Monaco in May, I hit a (figurative) wall. I stopped progressing, and I felt like I was running as fast as I could but going nowhere. It was affecting me on the race track, physically and mentally. Racing is a mental sport—yes, it's very tough physically, but it also takes a lot of mental skill to consistently do the same thing lap after lap.

I eventually went to the doctor for an unrelated problem, just a skin rash. The doctor gave me some cream and asked if there was anything else bothering me. I told him about my extreme thirst—I had been drinking seven or eight bottles of water every night, but it just never seemed like enough. He was jotting down notes and then asked me if I had lost any weight. Being an athlete, I had been training pretty hard and paying close attention to my nutrition, so I knew that I had lost some weight. When he put me on the scale, I couldn't believe that I had lost twenty-five pounds in one week. It was right then that I realized something was seriously wrong. The doctor told me that it was likely that I had type 1 diabetes.

I was in shock and disbelief. There I was, a professional athlete in otherwise good health, and all of a sudden I had a diagnosis that I honestly didn't understand at the time. I'll be the first to admit I was ignorant about all things diabetes. Type 1 diabetes does not run in my family, and I hadn't really been exposed to any friends with diabetes. So I went home from the doctor's office and researched everything I could online about diabetes. Frankly, I was overwhelmed.

Fortunately, my dad was flying into England that evening for my upcoming race. I picked him up from the bus station, and we went to dinner across the street. We sat down, ordered our meals, and I said to him, "Dad, I went to the doctor, and he thinks I have diabetes." Then I burst into tears.

The next day my dad and I went to an endocrinologist at Oxford University and eventually asked the one question that had been on my mind since I stepped on the scale the day before: "Will I still be able to race?" It seemed like a lifetime before the doctor answered, though I'm sure it was seconds. He casually looked up and said, "I don't see why not. There are amazing people with diabetes doing amazing things every day."

From that moment on, it felt like a weight had been lifted. I was still overwhelmed—obviously my life was going to change. But I quickly learned that I had a great support system behind me… from the expert doctors to my family, and especially the diabetes community as a whole. Because I needed some time to get back in shape and take control of the diabetes, I had to put racing on hold for the rest of the season—a tough decision, but an important one for sure. After a news release was sent out announcing my diagnosis, I received messages of support from people all over the world—China, Texas, Holland, and of course, home in California.

My world stopped spinning out of control at that point. I had a plan and a path toward getting back in a race car. I learned as much as I could about type 1 diabetes, so I had a better understanding of what was going on with my body. I worked with my doctor to find a treatment regimen that kept me healthy and strong, both on and off the race track. I took advantage of the time out of the race car to spend time with friends and family, mountain bike, and get out on the water. Getting stronger, physically and mentally, was just another step in preparing for the start of the next race season.

Thanks to my support system and a lot of hard work, I was back in a race car six months later in the Formula 3 Euroseries, and I earned a second place finish at my first race after my type 1 diabetes diagnosis. While standing up on the podium, it hit me—I am no different from who I was before my diagnosis. I'm still the same racing driver with the same skills and goals. It was honestly a relief to be able to prove this, not only to the racing world and to my doctors, but mainly to my toughest critic: myself. That podium finish gave me a ton of confidence to keep going for the win each race weekend and to move up to more challenging series as I gained more experience on the track.

From the Minor League to the Major League

In 2009, I returned to the United States to compete in the Firestone Indy Lights series. And, as they say, the rest is history. I began a groundbreaking partnership with the global diabetes care company, Novo Nordisk®. It started out and continues today as a true partnership—more than just a racing sponsorship. They make the insulins and the delivery devices that I use every day to manage my diabetes. We worked together to make pharmaceutical marketing history with the first pharmaceutical branded tweet (via our Twitter account @racewithinsulin). Later that year, I began traveling the country speaking on behalf of Novo Nordisk and sharing my story with others who have diabetes.

After two successful seasons in Firestone Indy Lights, I was fortunate to realize one of my dreams and move up to the IZOD IndyCar Series, the premier North American open-wheel racing series, with the newly-formed Novo Nordisk Chip Ganassi Racing team. To race under the Ganassi name is such an honor. I drive the Number 83 race car as a tribute to both Chip Ganassi and my dad. Not only was it the year of Chip Ganassi's career-best Indianapolis 500 finish as a racing driver, but it was also in a car that my father helped design.

In May of 2011, I lived another one of my dreams: racing in the historic Indianapolis 500. Words can't describe what it felt like to be introduced on the Yard of Bricks at the largest single-day sporting event in the world. I still get chills when I think about it! And being the first driver with diabetes to qualify and finish the race made the experience that much *sweeter* (no pun intended).

Racing with Diabetes and Realizing My Dream

Racing in Firestone Indy Lights, the final step in INDYCAR's developmental ladder program before the IZOD IndyCar Series, gave me an opportunity to really hone in on the best ways to make sure that I had my diabetes under control while on the track. At the race track, I wear a continuous glucose monitor that transmits to a receiver mounted in my race car. With this system, my blood sugar level is displayed on the steering wheel and transmitted back to my pit-timing stand where it is monitored by my engineer. This system allows my team and me to keep an eye on my sugar levels while racing.

If I'm burning off more glucose than expected, or if my numbers are falling more quickly than I anticipated, I have a drink tube in my helmet connected to a drink bottle filled with orange juice.

Now that I'm racing in the IZOD IndyCar Series, the racing events are a little longer and more strenuous than my previous races. Therefore, in addition to the drink tube, we also have an emergency insulin kit in the pit stand just in case it is needed. However, I've never even needed to use the orange juice during a race or open the emergency kit, which I credit to my doctors, training, and nutrition preparation.

While stepping out of my car after my first 500-mile race in 2011, I had a realization, similar to being on the podium at my first race after my diagnosis years earlier: there's absolutely nothing that I can't accomplish with diabetes. And the same goes for all of the people I meet with diabetes. I'm constantly overwhelmed and humbled by the response I receive at the race track and at appearances. The fan support and the courage of others I meet with diabetes inspires me to work even harder, not only as a racing driver but also as an athlete with diabetes.

Going back to October 16th, 2007, the date of my diagnosis, I was most worried that I'd never get back in a race car. Since that time, I've had to reevaluate what diabetes means to me as a person, as an athlete, and as a racing driver, and I'm stronger in each aspect of my life for that. Similar to race weekends, when I work with my engineers and crew for a fast car and good race result, I've had the support of family, friends, my medical team, fans and so many others to realize that there's nothing in life that I can't do with diabetes.

Though it may sound crazy, I truly see my diagnosis as a blessing in disguise. It has made me work harder than I thought I ever could, and I think the experiences I've had because of diabetes will help me both on and off track in the future. I'm in the fortunate position to do what I love—to drive race cars—but also to inspire and help people overcome challenges in managing diabetes and live their own passion. As I tell fans each race weekend, I'll never let diabetes slow me down.

www.CharlieKimball.com

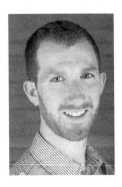

CHAPTER 12   *by Ken Kotch*

Picture This: A Photographer with a Broken Pancreas

One of my earliest memories is being at the pediatrician with my sister, Suzy (who is two years older), and fighting each other to see who could get deeper into the corner of the office to avoid getting a shot. At the time, I never felt as though I had won because, when we both left the doctor's office, we both had gotten a vaccination shot. If I had known then that shots would soon be part of my daily life, I wonder how much my behavior would have changed.

Diagnosis

Mom, Dad, Suzy, and I all had the flu. My brother was the only one who avoided it. Mom got better. Dad got better. Suzy got better. I got worse.

On Friday, Mom took me to the doctor, who said I didn't have strep or anything to worry about and sent me home. By Sunday, I started to feel better. Monday morning the tides turned again, so I stayed home from school. By lunch, I felt great and wondered why I wasn't in school. I went back to school for the rest of the week. Some days I felt okay, others not so much. But by the end of the week, I was struck with a constant thirst. I didn't care what I was drinking; I just wanted more.

My teachers started telling me that I could not go to the bathroom because I was asking to go two or three times in each class. Then I would go between classes and repeat the cycle. At home, Mom asked me why I was drinking so much. "I am thirsty," was my eight-year-old reply. Relieved that I had free reign of the bathroom at home, I planned to sleep in on Saturday morning. That never happened. Somewhere around 4 a.m., an uncomfortable feeling woke me up: I had wet my bed. That hadn't happened since I was in diapers.

I was afraid to awaken my parents to tell them, so I changed my pajamas and slept on the floor, embarrassed. By morning I had gotten up at least three times to urinate. The same thing happened for the next few nights, but this time I woke Mom to help me.

My mom asked me if I was eating all of my lunch at school. "Of course I am. I'm starving. Why?" Mom said that I looked as if I had lost weight. At that point, I had been sick for over two weeks. Mom took me back to my pediatrician for the third time. They took a urine sample and a blood test and sent me back to the waiting room. A few minutes later, we heard people shuffling around. Mom and I were the only ones there, so we knew it was for me. My doctor came out and told Mom to take me directly to the hospital where there were nurses waiting for me. The doctor said she hadn't ever seen such a colorful test strip. (Back in 1988, blood glucose was checked by matching the color of a strip to the side of a bottle. It would indicate what range the blood sugar was in.)

Hospital

Mom drove me to the hospital. Most of that day, November 23rd, 1988, and the next day are a blur. What I do remember is not very positive. Every time the nurses needed to check my blood sugar, they had to come in at least thirty minutes early to pry my hands apart to prick a finger. Eventually, I realized it was going to happen no matter what, so I stopped fighting. It was two days before Thanksgiving, and I had really been looking forward to having a few days off from school, hanging out with my friends, and having Thanksgiving dinner with my family. Instead, I was stuck in a hospital.

My first positive memory in the hospital was the delivery of my "Thanksgiving dinner." There was a roll, an apple, and a slice of dry turkey. The part that made me smile was the white rose towering over my lackluster meal. Something about that rose clicked and convinced me that everything was going to be okay. At that moment, I started to believe what my new endocrinologist, Dr. S., told me: "There is no reason that you shouldn't live to be one hundred, and there are only two things you shouldn't do: skydive and scuba dive. Those are the two things I wouldn't do, so I don't think you should either."

Of course, since then I have gone both skydiving and scuba diving.

I had lost more than 10% of my body weight, mostly through dehydration. Dr. S. said I looked like a wrinkled old man. I had two choices: either get an intravenous drip or drink a case of diet soda. Diet soda wasn't my idea of happiness, but it beat another needle. I didn't really care how much I was drinking; what I really wanted was to stack enough soda cans to block the door. Although I drank several cases, I never reached that goal.

On Monday, when my sister came to visit me, she brought get-well cards that the kids in my class had made for me. One from a boy in my class, Tommy, sticks in my mind. It was a piece of green construction paper folded in half with the words "Get Well Soon" written in marker on the front. Inside was a drawing of a kid (me) strapped to a stretcher with a nurse hovering over with a HUGE needle. The kid was yelling, "HELP!" My first thought was, *That is not what it's like. Shots don't bother me the way they did when I was younger."*

I found Tommy at recess on my first day back at school, and I told him that his picture had nothing to do with my life or diabetes. Tommy didn't hear, "We are lucky to have a simple way to test blood sugar at home." He didn't hear, "I am so glad it is 1988 and not before 1921, when the first human was injected with insulin." When my teacher explained to the class what was going on with me, all he heard was, "Ken has to take shots." I explained to him that everyone has an organ called the pancreas, and I had a "broken" pancreas. The part of mine that regulates the amount of sugar in my blood no longer worked. After that, and after seeing that I was still a faster runner, he started to understand that I wasn't going to let anything slow me down. Even though I had to plan things out a little more, I was still the same Ken.

The First Summer

My parents agreed that I was old enough to go to sleep-away camp that summer with my brother and sister. I dreamed about it every night. It was February or March when I realized that I couldn't go. I didn't yet know how to test my own blood sugar or take my own shot. I was devastated. Dr. S. suggested that I check out Camp Nejeda, a camp for kids with diabetes that was not far from where I lived. It was only two weeks instead of the four-week getaway with my siblings, but it was still a sleep-away camp.

In May that year, my parents took me to visit the camp and to see what it was all about. I fell in love immediately. Two minutes into my visit, I met the first person aside from me who had diabetes; Ira took me on a tour of the camp. He took me to the cabins, the archery range, the ropes course, the lake, and my favorite: the rocketry cabin. I was eight. The idea of building something, sending it into the sky, and blowing it up was right up my alley.

That July, when my parents dropped me off, I couldn't get them to leave soon enough. Seventy-five other kids with diabetes! Even some of the nurses had it. People without diabetes stuck out. My goals at camp were to learn to test my own blood sugar and to take my own shot. The deal was that, if I learned to do both of those things, my parents would buy me a skateboard: perfect motivation.

The first day at lunch, I saw the seven other kids and three counselors in my cabin testing their blood sugar. I was too shy to tell anyone that I had never done it. What was an eight-year-old to do? "Click." I pricked my finger and had a silent celebration in my head!

At dinner, I tested my blood sugar again. I was having so much fun that I didn't think twice about it. When the nurse got to our cabin to help load our syringes, I told her that I didn't know how to take a shot. She asked if I wanted to learn, and I said yes. So, before dinner on the first day, I had done two things that scared me the most. If that had been all I got from Camp Nejeda, that would have been more than enough. That night, I sent my mom a postcard. All it said was, "Get your checkbook ready. I'm getting a skateboard!"

Being able to talk with kids my age who had had the same experiences was a great comfort and a learning experience. Seeing counselors who were much older and healthy gave me confidence that I could be like them, too. Ira ended up being one of my counselors that summer. He taught me all about living with diabetes, going to college and, of equal importance, how to properly blow up a rocket. Ira and I have remained friends ever since. I've gone back to Camp Nejeda almost every summer since then, as have many of the lifelong friends that I made there. Camp Nejeda will always be a place that I call home.

When it was over, there were still two weeks left before my brother and sister got home from their camp, so Mom took me to Florida to visit my grandparents. With my newly-found confidence, I was taking all my own shots and checking my own blood sugars. I felt pretty lucky that I got to spend extra time with Grandma and Grandpa that Mike and Suzy didn't get.

Of course, before we went to Florida, I got my new skateboard.

Making a Difference

My parents were always going to different charity events and donating to different causes. I never saw the outcome, so it didn't really register as the kind of thing I should do. My first Halloween with diabetes was coming up. Previously, Halloween was my favorite holiday. That year, I learned an important lesson: it was not all about me. Not wanting me to miss out on the fun of trick-or-treating, my parents proposed that I go out with my friends and collect as much candy as I could in my Star Wars™ pillow case. When I got home, two things happened:

1. Mom and Dad gave me five cents for each piece of candy that I collected.
2. We donated the candy to kids who were not healthy enough to trick-or-treat, but who could have some candy.

Win-win. Being able to see the smiles that those kids—my own age—gave me was worth not having any candy. The $9.35 almost didn't matter (in 1989, that was a lot of money to a nine-year-old). This giving-to-others thing started to click. I continued to give my candy away until I stopped trick-or-treating.

Fast forward a decade: I attended college at Northeastern University in Boston. While in school, I started riding a bike everywhere and eventually started doing charity rides. The first one I did was a three-day ride to benefit local HIV/AIDS organizations. I raised over $3000. The knowledge that I could help people get food and much needed medicine just by riding my bike made it easy to ask my friends, family, and teachers to sponsor me.

Another win-win.

At some point after college, I stopped doing so many charity rides. Instead, I would write a check to friends when they asked me to sponsor their events. I missed being part of the driving force, though; I needed to find something new. Before long, it found me.

I was in a coffee shop in downtown Boston having a cup of coffee and a warm chocolate chip cookie. I had taken a *bolus* and everything was running smoothly until an acquaintance came up to me yelling, "You are going to kill yourself with that! You can't eat that!" These weren't new things, but something about that day made it different. It occurred to me that I had to do something to change the perception of diabetes.

As a photographer, I had always wanted to publish a book and, out of that coffee shop came the idea: Not only would I make great photographs of people living with diabetes, but I would also inspire those who weren't sure that they could achieve their goals. I came up with two rules for the people I would photograph:

1. You have to have diabetes. Any type will do.
2. You can't let it stop you from living your dreams.

It turned out that a lot of people fit those criteria. I started raising money and planning my trip. I would travel around the United States for a month and photograph twenty-five people, but first I needed a name for my project. Sitting with my friends, Robyn and Mandy, and brainstorming names, I threw out a few terrible ideas, and one of them asked me to clarify what diabetes is. I explained, just as I had when I was in third grade, that everyone has a pancreas. Part of mine is "broken" and doesn't make insulin. I get around it by taking insulin injections or wearing an insulin pump.

Robyn looked at me and said, "You have your name… Broken Pancreas."

With that taken care of, I needed to get funding and find subjects to photograph. I started a Facebook page called the Broken Pancreas Project. Within three days, I had 350 "likes." A week later, it was well over 500 (at the time of writing this chapter, we are approaching 1500). Forty-five days later, successful fundraising yielded the project a little more than $8000.

I rented a car and started driving on July 5, not to return home until the first week of August. I photographed over thirty people and drove more than 4000 miles. Even more exciting was that, while I drove, more and more people were joining the Facebook page and posting things like, "My pancreas broke on December 13th" or "I have a broken pancreas, too." The more I drove, the bigger the membership got. People started asking questions and looking for advice. It was becoming clear that Broken Pancreas should be more than just a book.

A few months after I got home from shooting, I re-defined the goals of Broken Pancreas. Broken Pancreas would be an educational organization. We will define what diabetes is and what it isn't. We will build a program to take into schools to teach these things to kids and to stop the stereotypes before they start (and throw in some tips on healthy living while we're at it). We will review diabetes products so People with Diabetes (PWDs) and their families can make more informed decisions about what will work best for them. We will inspire PWDs never to settle for ordinary.

The goal is to raise enough money each year to do all this and to send a few kids to diabetes camps for a crash course in living confidently with diabetes. We applied to become a 501(c)(3) non-profit organization and, through a lot of hard work and more volunteer hours from our attorney than I can count, we were accepted six months later. (For further information about my photography and the book, please see the website at the conclusion of this chapter.)

Learning to Speak up at School

I was diagnosed with diabetes in third grade. By fifth grade, I thought I had everything about diabetes figured out until my reading teacher, Mr. S., decided differently. Every day at 3 p.m., I had to leave the room, go to the nurse's office, and get a snack. Why I didn't just keep it in my desk eludes me now, but that is beside the point. Being a ten-year-old boy, I liked to sit in the back near the window so I could "fly under the radar"" and stare out the window to think about things greater than "Anne of Green Gables."

Because of diabetes and my need for a snack, Mr. S. mandated that I sit in the front corner right next to the door, so I wouldn't disturb the class when I got up to leave. As a class, we changed our seats about every month, except for me, stuck in the front corner. In the winter, our social studies class started studying discrimination. After that lesson, I realized that I had found my way out of the corner seat. One day after reading class, I went up to Mr. S. to ask about moving to a different seat the next time the class reorganized. I told him that he was discriminating against me because I had diabetes and, in a free society, that was not right.

He said he would think about it.

Now I don't know whether he took what I said to heart or if he was afraid of my mom (I was the last of her three children to go through the school, and Mom wasn't shy about standing up for us). I like to think that he took my carefully prepared, then stumbled-over, speech into consideration. The next time we chose new seats, he quietly let me know that I didn't have to sit by the door anymore. That was the last time I let someone else's thoughts determine my place, diabetes-related or not.

Colorblind

Before becoming a professional photographer, I went to Northeastern University to earn an Art degree with a concentration in Photography. Most of my professors could not have encouraged me more. There was one, however, who decided to take the opposite approach. Let's call him "Larry."

At the time, Larry taught Introduction to Color Photography, a prerequisite for moving on to more advanced classes. On the first day of class, I walked up to Larry and said, "I am red/green colorblind. This is not an excuse; I just thought I would let you know, so if my prints are way off, you will know why. If and when my colors are off, I hope you will allow me to correct them."

His response: "You should drop this class. You will never be able to pass."

Larry then told me I should choose a new major. I was still young and had time to reconsider my options.

I could not keep track of the number of times I had been told that I couldn't do things. The surprise here was that, this time, it wasn't diabetes-related. Having had so much practice succeeding where others said I could not definitely gave me an advantage in Larry's class. For me, walking away was not an option, and I thank diabetes for that.

Of course I stayed in the class—sometimes struggling—and earned an "A." The irony is that most of my favorite work today features very strong colors and is strongly related to the theories that I learned in that class. Was it easy? No. But anything worth doing is worth breaking your back for.

Photographer

I have found that diabetes is much easier to control when I live with a consistent schedule. Life as a photographer is anything but consistent. Some weeks I'm in my office and in meetings all week. Some weeks I'm running from job to job with no time for lunch, or shooting for nine hours straight with no time to treat low blood sugar.

Early in my career, when I was assisting other photographers, I never knew when or if we would take a lunch break. It forced me to be much more in tune with what my body was telling me. I am at a point now where I can live for about sixteen hours on no more than a granola bar and a pack of fruit snacks, which are a permanent part of my camera bag, pockets, car, etc. Always being prepared for long shoots has made my photography career easier to navigate. Before every shoot, I go through all of my gear to make sure that I have everything I could possibly need for the job, so that when the time comes, there are no surprises.

World

I'm often surprised by the continuing misinformation and stereotypes that PWDs encounter in the U.S.; it can sometimes be a struggle to get people to understand what diabetes is and what my needs are. Although I knew that it would be harder to communicate about my diabetes while living abroad, I still decided I should move to China.

I lived at a boarding school teaching English to students ages six to nineteen years old. The village down the street from the school had no running water and not much electricity. Not only did they have no concept of what diabetes was, for most of them, I was the first Caucasian person they had ever talked to. Add to that, when I landed there, I spoke a total of three words of Mandarin.

I lived in a suburb of Xi'an, a few hours' drive from where the Terracotta Warriors were found in 1974. Xi'an is regarded as the birthplace of the dumpling. For the first few days, I had no idea what I was eating, what it was cooked in, or how it would affect my blood sugar. All the years of "guesstimating" how many carbohydrates were in my food prepared me to do a pretty good job. After a week, I had dumplings down to a science. A standard fried dumpling was seven grams of carbohydrates; breaded dumplings were about eleven grams. Of course, depending on what kind of oil they were cooked in, the size of the dumpling, and what was in them, those numbers could shift as much as 50%. To make things easier, I lived on a very strict schedule. Meals were almost always at exactly the same time, which made planning much less difficult.

A few years later, when I moved to Florence, Italy, for half a year, I didn't think twice about food or how I would deal with controlling diabetes. At least this time, I could translate what each food was (which is tough to do when you don't know all the Chinese symbols).

I really feel that I could be dropped anywhere in the world now and figure out how to get by. That was China's gift to me. There was no one to ask, so I had to figure it out on my own.

Struggle

I am generally a pretty positive person. It is tough to offend me or to get me down. That said, diabetes can still be a struggle even after all these years. Sometimes I do everything "right," and it seems that my body doesn't listen to reason.

As I write this chapter, I am training to run (with my charity team) in the ING NYC Marathon. I haven't run a race since I was in sixth grade, but I've been riding my bike long distances for years, so I figured that managing my diabetes and running couldn't be that much different.

Not so.

On my bike, thirty-five to forty carbohydrates an hour is plenty to keep my blood sugar level in a safe target range. But when I'm running, it doesn't even scratch the surface. There are days when I prepare for a run and my body stops me in my tracks. My typical routine is to reduce my pump's *basal* rate to 3% an hour before I start and eat about forty-five grams of carbohydrates with some protein. Most days, that will get me through the first two miles before I have to start drinking double-strength Gatorade® and eating more.

One of the most valuable lessons I learned from Nurse Nancy at Camp Nejeda is that, even when you follow all the rules, sometimes things don't go according to plan. The reason? Sometimes it's just "because." I find it most frustrating when I cannot figure out why the blood sugar numbers are not matching what I think they should be. At those times, I remember what Nancy taught me: blood sugar numbers are a gauge, not a test score. They tell you where you are and where you were, and they help you make decisions on what to do next.

Advantages

Not many people would say this, but I am almost glad that I got diabetes. It is not who I am, but it helped to shape the person who I became. I've also found some perks.

One of my favorite desserts as a kid was an ice cream float. Before insulin pumps or *Lantus*® was available, I took NPH insulin (long acting). Every morning, I took forty-two units, and at night I took sixteen units. Mom usually loaded my shot for me, but one night she wasn't home, so Dad helped me out. Somehow, he switched my dose and accidentally gave me forty-two units right before bedtime. Realizing his mistake, he immediately called Dr. S., who calmly told my dad to make me a *big* ice cream float with regular soda and test me every hour overnight. I was in heaven, even though Dad had to deal with testing my blood sugar all night. He and Mom fed me when my blood sugar dropped low, but I slept right through it. Overall: Best dessert ever!

I am much more aware of the food that I put into my body than are my friends who live without diabetes. I have had to pay attention for more than two decades, and it is part of my life now. You can place any food in front of me, and I can tell you with absolute certainty how many grams of carbohydrate are in it and how it will affect my blood sugar and energy level. At a young age, I realized how much more energy I had and how much better I felt when I ate healthy food. Even though I love a good chocolate bar, I would rather have an apple.

Over the years, I have met people of all ages with diabetes. Some of them were diagnosed at a few months old, some a few years old, some in college, and some at retirement. If I had to get diabetes, I am glad it happened when I was eight years old. I was old enough to verbalize how I was feeling and take ownership of the disease. My parents weren't left guessing when my blood sugar was low because I was able to speak up.

By the time I left home to go to college, taking insulin, counting carbohydrates, and checking my blood sugar were as ingrained into my life as tying my shoes before leaving the house. I have known a number of people who were diagnosed with diabetes in high school. From my viewpoint, that is one of the hardest times to get diabetes. You are old enough to have set routines and are just becoming independent, when overnight you have to start learning all over. Of course, the people I knew who developed diabetes in high school thought the exact opposite. They couldn't imagine being diagnosed at a younger age.

At whatever age diabetes starts, there are two roads you can take:

1. This sucks. Why me?
2. This sucks. Here are the tools I have. I'm not slowing down!

I continue to choose the latter every day.

www.kenkotch.com

www.BrokenPancreas.org

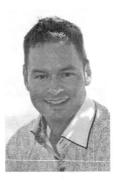

CHAPTER 13   *by Martin Lafontaine*

Living With Type 1 Diabetes: A 'Life PhD' to Success

A Few Words About Myself

First, for those who are wondering how to pronounce my first name with the right accent, don't worry. Any way you manage it while giving an honest try is great. But, if you insist on trying the French Canadian way, simply replace the "in" with "hein" and you should sound like a perfect French Canadian. So now give it your best shot… "Martein"! Not easy, eh? But thanks for trying.

Considered by many as the prototypical "corporate athlete," since business takes me around the world, I am more often on a plane and in a hotel than at home and in my own bed. I have been working for the past fourteen years of my young professional career in the pharmaceutical and medical device industry, building a broad expertise in the area of commercial launch excellence, organizational development, and business development, as well as in overall business management, in various business dynamic and cultural environments. Some people know me as a "philanthropic entrepreneur" too, having spent time in a South African township to inspire youth and to create hope and belief in a better future. Others could also associate me as the president and co-owner of a car racing team, which helps to occupy my otherwise free time. But to all, I want to be known first as this person who dedicates his time to the diabetes community to help move—or should I say remove—the needles one at a time. In a nutshell, I am a positive, forward-looking, glass-half-full, solution-oriented, striving individual who—using these life skills and positive attitude that living with type 1 diabetes has provided me—lives my life as a "successful man with diabetes." Living with type 1 diabetes CAN be the best tool one can have to live a happy, VERY successful, no-limits life. Living with type 1 diabetes has not limited my ability to achieve my goals, and it has assuredly not limited my capacity to dream new ones. Quite the opposite, actually, in that living with type 1 diabetes has been guiding my life to this very day.

This chapter will highlight what I feel were some of the best "courses" that I followed in the last twenty-five years of my life since being diagnosed with type 1 diabetes. I like to call it my "Life PhD." These will include "courses" from both my undergraduate lessons, such as "Diabetes 101: Why me?" to my graduate studies such as "Diabetes 201: You should not..." as well as some highlights on my post-graduate "Thesis: Respect to Diabetes." (Hmmm. I wonder if I will ever graduate.) I do hope that it will challenge some perceptions and views, as well as the relationships, that people living with type 1 diabetes might have with the condition.

So let's get going by first having a quick look at the very first days.

My First Date with Type 1 Diabetes

I was lying in my parents' bed, at 2:58 p.m. I had been through a day-long series of doctor appointments and tests and was now anxiously waiting to get the final word on what had been "wrong" with me for the past few weeks. In school, I had become a nuisance to both my classmates and teacher, asking to go to the bathroom every five minutes or so! And what about my repeated trips to the water fountain? Apart from that, all seemed okay; except for the color change on an old test strip that Mom had me urinate on that morning. But those were old strips she had had for so long that she wasn't worried too much about their suggested verdict.

Then, the expected 3 p.m. phone call from the doctor suddenly rang. The long wait was about to come to an end. But I didn't have time to be sick. I had hockey practice to get ready for and two important hockey games coming up that weekend. And you know how important hockey is to us Canadians!!! But then again, I had been off from school all day, which made the whole thing rather fun, actually.

What I remember most of that fateful phone call was hearing Mom pick up the phone after not even half a ring, and fifteen seconds later, I heard her falling in tears. Mom did not cry easily. That was when I knew something bad had happened to me, and that it might be bad enough for me to miss the evening's hockey practice.

It was at that moment that I decided to jump out of bed to join my parents in the living room and ask them what was happening…to me. That moment has stayed engraved in my memory for all of my life. Mom was unable to speak; she was crying and crying, repeatedly asking, "*pourquoi?*" (Why?) My dad, Serge, tried to calm Mom to the best of his abilities, and from my recollection, he wasn't very successful at that. (Sorry, Dad.) And then they saw me coming towards them.

"*Qu'est-ce que c'est? Qu'est-ce que j'ai?*" I asked. (What is it? What do I have?)

Neither of them responded, but the expression on their faces said it all. After looking down for a moment (I would guess to muster up the courage needed to face me), Dad said, with a broken voice, "Everything will be fine, Son. Everything will be okay. Let's go and pack up your luggage, and bring your pajamas."

As the stress and anxiety rose inside me, the tone of my voice changed: "What do I have, Dad? Can I still go to my practice tonight? We're playing two important games this weekend, and I must get ready for them…. Dad, you of all people should know how important these games are!"

You can well imagine that I didn't make my hockey practice that night.

Only once, when I sat facing the doctor at the hospital, was I told what was happening to me. "You have diabetes," he said, in answer to the same question I repeatedly asked Mom and Dad at home and all the way to the hospital.

"I have diabetes? Isn't that a disease that old people have?" (It didn't make sense; it couldn't be happening to someone who was only thirteen years old at the time. Granted, I was a very mature thirteen years old, but still…?)

"Okay Doc, I have diabetes. But will I be able to play hockey this weekend?" I asked hopefully. "It'll be okay if I miss the practice tonight; I'm ready for those games anyway…." I added. With hindsight, I recognize that this was a very child-like response, which was normal you will say, right? But I'll refer again to this childish attitude later on in the chapter and to the importance of keeping it alive and well, somehow, throughout our lives living with type 1 diabetes.

The doctor then went on to explain that my body was no longer able to produce that hormone called insulin and that from then on, I would have to be careful not to eat too much sugar. "Oh no! And what about Nutella®? And my favorite cereals?" Now this was the toughest part! Or so I thought… until the doctor continued by adding that I would have to give myself… SHOTS!

"What!!! Give myself shots? Dad, is that true?"

That did not sound very cool to me. But the doctor was patient and helped me understand that I didn't have a choice. What my body couldn't produce, I had to supply with shots. Okay, I thought, not the most pleasant notion, but then again, he was the one wearing the white coat, so he must know what he's talking about! And if he said I must, then I guess I had to.

As I sat there, I recalled that I had had blood tests done before, and they hadn't been so very bad. I turned to Dad and asked, "Fine with the shots, but how long will I have to do this?" I figured that I could take this for a while, but how long will it have to be? There was dead silence in the room. No answer.

With a little more nervousness in my voice, I asked again: "But Dad, how long will I have to do this, tell me. How long?" My father remained silent, as did my mother. And both of their expressions looked gloomy. The situation didn't sound good to me. Not a good sign! With as much insistence as I could dare use for my age, I asked for a third time: "Dad, HOW LONG? Please, tell me. Please!"

Then, as hard as it must have been for him, he finally answered me: "Five to ten years, my Son, maybe less." I noticed a calendar on the wall. November 24, 1987. I mentally flipped five years of pages. November 24, 1992. At least it wouldn't be forever....

My dad recalled the doctors telling him back on that fateful day that a cure would most likely be found within five years. So he gave me hope while the medical community figured out how to cure me. I would never blame my parents for the answers they gave me. All they were doing was telling me what they themselves were told and put their hope in. How were they to know that no cure would be forthcoming five years later? Or, for that matter ten years later, or....

One thing I've learned in my professional career from older, wiser businessmen is that the one asking the better questions often ends up better off than the one who thinks he or she knows all the better answers. So on that day of November 24, 1987, with that in mind, what if I were the one not asking the right question? Just a thought...

Diabetes 101: "Why Me?"

I was diagnosed with type 1 diabetes during that very troublesome period of life called adolescence, characterized by an increased desire for independence and autonomy. But we all know that there's a lot more to adolescence than just that: hormonal changes of all kinds, a sudden desire to "be cool," to fit in with peers, and so much more. And perhaps most important of all to an adolescent is the need to conform—all qualities that might not always, at first glance, be a good match with a diagnosis of type 1 diabetes.

Throughout my school years, I was considered a pretty popular guy. I was always surrounded by an amazing group of close friends that I could count on when needed and I can also claim a fair bit of success with the ladies (which I hope will last forever!). I was a top performing student and athlete, winning awards year after year. I was considered a great prospect for professional hockey, being awarded Best Hockey Goaltender in Canada at the age of fourteen. Between my friends, my academic success, my athletic prowess, and, ahem, the ladies, one would say that I had it made!

The next few years were terrific. I was always getting great summer jobs, and I completed a Bachelor of Science degree in Medical Biology, finishing first in my class. I was offered many jobs upon graduation including offers of post-graduate studies. I should have felt lucky to have all this success, and what seemed like a prolific future to which to look forward. But something wasn't quite right. Two little words stuck in the back of my head, keeping me from appreciating all these achievements.

From the announcement of my diagnosis at the Hospital in *Trois-Rivieres*, and despite the good care I had been providing to myself since then, I subconsciously had permitted the question "Why me?" to hold me back from fully seeing myself as the successful individual that I was. I felt different from everybody else. Having diabetes somehow meant that there was something weak, incorrect about me. So in response to this, I shied away from letting anyone know about my difference, see my difference, or share my concerns about my "perceived weaknesses." After all, teenagers buy tons of products and will do just about anything to hide a simple pimple, right? Well, when it came to my diabetes, that was true for me until the day....

On that fateful summer night, I had dinner at a restaurant in my hometown of *Trois-Rivieres*, Québec, with my great childhood friend Sébastien Vouligny (whom we called Voul for short). Today a very successful professional life coach, Sébastien was sharing with me his views on how particular events in our past help to forge what we become later in life; moreover, how these events help us grow as human beings in general. Just before dinner arrived, I got up and walked to the bathroom (read: the closest hidden place) to test my blood glucose and give my needed insulin dose, making sure that no one saw "my difference." Back at the table, Sébastien asked me where I had just been.

"I went to the bathroom Voul, you know, to test my blood glucose and give my shot as I always do before a meal."

Sébastien didn't reply, but instead put his utensils down and said: "Okay. I need you to explain something to me. In fact, I really need you to help me understand something."

"No problem, Voul. What can I help you with, buddy?"

I will never forget the ninety seconds that followed. What was said next was a real eye opener for me, and I honestly believe should be read by all who live with type 1 diabetes, or have faced lifelong challenges of any kind, for that matter.

"There is something I don't get about you Martin," Sébastien said. "You're a very successful guy. You have done well in school, collecting awards year after year. You've been a top athlete at hockey and good at many other sports. You're having a great professional career on the go. Ladies like you. People like being around you, and you've been an inspiration to us all through your life discipline, resiliency, and continuous search to surpass yourself. With all this behind you, and achievements surely to come, you must be very proud of yourself, right?"

"Uh, yes I am, Voul. I guess I am, thanks buddy. I appreciate your saying that."

"Well then, am I also right in saying that most likely, your diabetes diagnosis at age thirteen has been one, if not the key event of your life, thus far?" Sébastien added.

"Yup, definitely. It's 24/7 for me Voul, so it has to be," nodding positively again.

"So then, if you're proud of who you've become to this day, and that, as you said, your diabetes diagnosis was surely the key event in your life, so far, and that, as you said, is part of your everyday life, 24/7, then wouldn't you think this has something to do with who you are now; that your diabetes has provided ample daily opportunity to practice multiple life skills such as discipline, rigor, hard work, will power, resiliency, and also positivism, that helped you become that person you are today? Would that make any sense at all?"

As I was looking silently at Sébastien, he added, "And now, by hiding in the bathroom to test your blood sugars and give yourself a shot, it strikes me that you are hiding probably the most important contributor to your success, to the amazing person that you are today with all those key skills and attitudes. Skills and attitudes that will help you keep going in life, whatever you choose to do! Help me here. I am sorry, but I simply don't get it!"

That ninety-second chat with Sébastien forever changed my world and gave me a whole new perspective on my relationship with diabetes. Instead of looking at diabetes as a barrier to contend with, it was that situation that gave me the needed skills to strive for a productive and successful life! One doesn't achieve success *despite* living with type 1 diabetes; one achieves success in part *due to* living with diabetes and all the life skills practiced, learned, and acquired as a result. My "defective pancreas" actually became the catalyst to help me gain more strength and the ability to practice and acquire a successful "Life PhD"! To use the words of a good friend and mentor, Dr. William (Bill) Polonsky, I had my "something clicked" moment.

My "Diabetes 101 course: Why me?" taught me that, behind every setback resides an opportunity: the tougher the setback, the bigger the opportunity. Whenever I think about some setback that I have faced in my life, I have to thank my diabetes. There was that job that I applied for early on in my professional career and did not get, but that actually turned out to be my chance to go on a new path that would drive my professional development to a whole new level. And there was that painful heartbreak in my late twenties that ended up becoming an opportunity to realign the direction I wanted to give to my life and live my craziest dreams. I have to thank my type 1 diabetes to have equipped me with this positive, forward-looking attitude that helped turn obstacles into opportunities with even more positive outcomes. Therefore, in the absence of a good answer to the profound question "Why me?" in all these years, I guess the only possible answer I could come up with is "Why not me?!"

Diabetes 201: "You Should Not..."

As I mentioned before, where I'm from (the province of Québec, Canada) and, for that matter, pretty well everywhere in Canada, hockey is practically a religion. One of—if not the most—celebrated heroes that the sport produced, Wayne Gretzky, once said: "You miss 100% of the shots you don't try." I have always found this statement extremely powerful and a great motto for resilience.

Sadly, one of the few things I do remember when I was first told that I had type 1 diabetes was that, from then on, there would be some things that I could not do anymore, or that I should not do, due to my "new condition." I was a very active kid in a discovery mode, and those warnings rocked my little world. To my dismay, this would have to be my fate for at least the forecasted five years, or who knows, maybe even longer! It's one thing for someone to consciously limit oneself, but something else when you feel the world has opened up for you and now you are being told to limit, reduce, minimize, or worse—"don't even think about it!"

Throughout my adolescence and early adulthood, I couldn't count the number of times, because of me having diabetes, that my parents and I were served the "He should not...." or "He won't be able to because...." Many people simply found it easier to assume that I could not do something rather than actually inquiring about what I could or could not do. I wouldn't want to blame anyone. All those teachers, trainers, managers and so forth were probably scared or lacked insight to diabetes, and did what they did with good intentions. But, by their limiting actions, they made matters worse. I remember playing a hockey game in *Sorel* (Québec), with my dad watching me from the stands (he never missed a game). Dad became furious and felt rage building inside him as he overheard a few scouts discuss the case of "this young talented Lafontaine, a goaltender, so good and fast, but having diabetes, therefore, probably won't have the strength required to play a full season in the big league." My dad was usually a calm guy, but that day at the arena, he became understandably furious as he bore witness to the misperceptions that people had about type 1 diabetes and its impact on his son. Or, more recently, I had to face a similar situation in an interview, when I was asked if I would be able to handle all the travel required for that job, "because...you know...your condition." I chose to share these two stories with you, but believe me, I could have given you more; the list goes on and on.

If we listened to what some people say and think, type 1 diabetes could be a limiting factor that could make us half-successful or half-happy in life. I've researched many pages of scientific literature on diabetes over the years, and nowhere have I found that living with type 1 diabetes means that people must limit themselves to live half-happy, half-productive, or half-successful lives.

Remember when I said earlier in this chapter that staying "childish" throughout our lives with type 1 diabetes is essential? For most of us, when our parents said we weren't allowed to do something, the natural reaction was to give it a try! Right? To make our own experiences and to learn. And yes, we learn from the good shots and the not-so-good shots. Therefore, I have lived my life with the opposition of a child, always, by pushing back on the limits that others have imposed on me "because of my condition." And I find it infinitely more appealing to find out how far I can go instead of how long my chain is! Don't you?

Because of this rebel-like attitude, notwithstanding my diabetes, I:

- Moved away from home at age sixteen, not only with my bags, but also with Mom and Dad's trust, in order to pursue my dream of playing my sport at the highest level—only a little more than two years after sharing my life with "Miss Needle";
- Have been at super university parties that I somewhat remember… partially, and survived (Oops. Sorry, Mom.);
- Played ice hockey at a highly competitive level, believing that I was strong enough to last a whole season and therefore benefiting from the competitive and teamwork skills that playing team sports gave, alongside that desire for continuous improvement and a winning attitude;
- Moved to the English speaking part of Canada early on in my professional career (not speaking the language) to take on a marketing position with my employer, despite my lack of knowledge in this area. (I had earned a Bachelor of Science degree in Medical Biology and taken a unique business course, Introduction to Marketing 101). That led me to occupy a global marketing leadership role within my corporation years later;
- Travelled around the world for business, flying more than 100 times a year while eating out five days a week because I thought I could find a way to eat responsibly and compensate for different time zones and therefore, live my passion and realize another one of my crazy dreams;
- Worked six months in a South African slum, leaving by myself with my bags and the courage to launch a new model of excellence in the care of orphans and vulnerable children. This new model was based on community empowerment and on building the sense of BELIEF and hope that things can change for a better future. And yes, they are changing…

So, throughout my life living with type 1 diabetes, I've been pushing my limits, living life at 110%, often out-distancing people with working pancreases, following my most crazy dreams, while finding diabetes to be an enabler that drives me forward rather than a barrier to break my stride. I do all of this while being respectful of my diabetes, always factoring in what should be done to prevent problems by thinking ahead. And I can say with absolute honesty that my parents' empowering and trusting attitudes paved the road to where I am today. And for dessert (figuratively speaking, that is), I'm able to boast an A1c consistently between 7% and 7.5% over all these years.

Now, to those who, in the past, have tried to stop me in my tracks, I say, "Thank you very much!" You are partially responsible for my success, giving me the inspiration to push forward instead of listening to your well-meaning yet limiting advice. As William Arthur Ward, well known for his inspirational quotes, once said: "Adversity causes some men to break; others to break records."

The challenge of living with type 1 diabetes should be looked at the same way. I challenge you, the reader, to take the steps to make your own "crazy dreams" happen.

My "Respect to Diabetes" Thesis

Type 1 diabetes, despite having added a lot of work, frustration, and several dates at 3 a.m. with my refrigerator over the last twenty-five years, has taught me a lot. I am a guy who values respect. I believe in being fair in life. Therefore, if I am being true to myself, and believe that living with type 1 diabetes has given me so many opportunities over the years to grow, to become the person who I am today, and living a happy and productive no-limits life, then I do owe diabetes respect and have to be grateful for it.

Due to my philanthropic nature, I want to give back to diabetes. First and most importantly, giving back to my own diabetes. I try my best and work hard at sustaining my efforts to focus on the "controllable" in order to keep my blood glucose within the desired range and let go of the rest. I need to respect my own diabetes since, as we all know, *uncontrolled* diabetes can bring us some unpleasant surprises; I repeat, UNCONTROLLED diabetes. And I need to be conscious of that and take care of it! After all, it just makes sense to take care of myself.

Second, giving back to people just like me, living with type 1 diabetes and going through similar struggles, is also very important. And to this regard, I would like to acknowledge the support of a very important person in my life— my personal coach, Denise Caissie, who has been instrumental in many ways. One way she helps me is by constantly encouraging and working with me to leverage my skills and attitudes, broadening my impact in helping and giving back to people who are living with diabetes. Denise, a big thank you!

Over the years, I have joined several organizations that aim to support people living with diabetes to live healthy and productive lives. One of those is the Behavioral Diabetes Institute (BDI) in San Diego, California, founded by Dr. William Polonsky and Dr. Susan Guzman. The BDI is the world's first organization dedicated to tackling the unmet psychological needs of people with diabetes. I first met Dr. Polonsky in 2005 at the Canadian Diabetes Conference in Edmonton, where he gave a talk on the psychosocial impact of living with diabetes. I was truly amazed by his talk, and I wanted to dedicate my efforts to the emotional and psychosocial sides of living with type 1 diabetes, since it is so critical to all patients and families living with type 1 diabetes, but at the same time is so under-served. I joined the Board of Directors of the BDI shortly after, and my role now, in line with my skills and expertise, is to develop international partnerships to help increase the reach and impact of the Institute and its unique offering to patients, families, healthcare professionals, and other key stakeholders involved in the care and support of people living with diabetes. (For further information about the Behavioral Diabetes Institute, please see their website listed at the conclusion of this chapter.)

Another organization that I give my time to is American Youth Understanding of Diabetes Abroad (AYUDA). It is a volunteer-based organization in which youth serve as agents of change, dedicated to working with local diabetes communities to develop and implement sustainable diabetes programs throughout the world. AYUDA is an amazing organization founded in 1996 by Dr. Nic Cuttriss, who was just fifteen years old at the time. I joined the Board of Directors of AYUDA in 2010. (For more information about AYUDA, please see their website listed at the conclusion of this chapter.)

I also recently served as a faculty member for the International Diabetes Federation (IDF) Young Leaders in Diabetes Programme, a group of over sixty like-minded young leaders from all over the world, united with one single mission: enhancing the lives of young people living with diabetes. Being part of the Young Leader's faculty gave me the chance to meet and interact with a group of amazing young people in the international diabetes community.

And I have also recently played a leadership role in bringing an innovative treatment option to Canadian patients living with type 1 diabetes, while building the required infrastructure to provide its access to patients and now directing the commercial operations.

Thirdly and finally, I also believe that giving back to the ones who have been there all along the way is essential, and this includes my friends, girlfriends, medical team members (special note to my family doctor, Dr. Fernand Paille from *Trois-Rivieres*), and to my family. I dedicate this chapter to my mom and dad, Serge and Lorraine, who have, without any prior lessons or preparation, been the best parents a child with diabetes could ever have. Mom, Dad: you have been instrumental in allowing me to live my life to the fullest and to graduate with a "Life PhD." Mom, Dad…"*Merci pour tout!*" Also, thanks to my brother, Patrick, who, despite not having to inject himself every day, surely felt the impact of my diagnosis, indirectly.

It's strange, sometimes, the curve balls that life throws at us. In the last five years, both my mom and my dad were diagnosed with type 2 diabetes. Giving back to diabetes in this situation took on a whole new meaning, and it could not hit any closer to home. My mom's reaction to her diagnosis, and shortly thereafter having to start on insulin injections, wasn't as bad as one might think. Why so? I have tried to find the answer to this question for years, so far unsuccessfully. Maybe because it was a way for her to experience and live through what her little boy had to do and live with all these years? Or maybe it was a way for her to take on some of that pain from her little boy? Mom always had a difficult time watching me inject myself, as if she felt the needle herself. You can imagine the smile on my face the first time that Mom and I sat side by side at the dinner table and took our respective insulin pens to give ourselves our shots. No, I did not go to the bathroom that time. And then my mom told me, with her amazing smile, "You were right. It does not hurt."

My dad responded very differently to his diagnosis. It was a shock to him. I will always remember the day that Dad and I were speaking at home following his diagnosis, talking about blood sugar testing and other things related to what diabetes management would mean for him. At some point in our discussion, I felt that I had to ask Dad how he felt about all this: the diet, the blood glucose testing, and the exercise regimen that he had to start, amongst other things. It seemed like it would be a lot for him to take on board, despite his knowledge of diabetes, as per his son's experience. He told me that it seemed like "*déjà vu*," except that this time, the roles were reversed.

"So, Dad. How are things? How are you dealing with all of this?" I asked, as he sat at the table, his head down. He slowly raised his head and, with a convincing and reassuring tone, told me, "It will all be okay, my Son. It will all be okay." A few words that sounded very familiar….

Let's Catch the Opportunity… Now!

I don't wish diabetes for anyone. Let's be clear on this. And diabetes is not fun: no doubt about that. But, like every curve ball or challenge thrown at us in life, there are always two ways to look at it: the glass being half-empty or the glass being half-full. And this attitude we take in facing those curve balls and challenges is 100% part of the "controllable."

I am also from the school of thought that hard work pays dividends. Mom was raised on the farm, so I guess I owe that to her. And yes, diabetes is a lot of hard work. And true, the efforts of good diabetes management can help us avoid some of the potential complications that can be associated with this disease, which is, in itself, a major reward for our hard work. But the reward from living well with type 1 diabetes can be a whole lot more.

Living with type 1 diabetes can provide us with a "Life PhD" in itself. A "PhD" that provides its rigorous and disciplined students a set of key skills, attitudes, and knowledge that can lead them through very productive, healthy, no-limits lives that can out-pace people living with healthy pancreases. True, it's a very demanding degree, requiring lots of effort and homework, but one that can set you up for your dream job!

Going back to the day of November 24, 1987 and Dad's response to my 'How long?' question, I realized with time that perhaps I did not ask the right question. Had I known way back when I was diagnosed with type 1 diabetes what I know now, I would have questioned my dad differently. On that day, maybe I should have asked my father, "Dad, how long will it take me to realize that living with type 1 diabetes will provide me with the life skills, strengths, and ability to strive for whatever I want in life, and achieve it?" To this question, dad's answer would have been right.

So, to all my fellow diabetes brothers and sisters living with type 1 diabetes: let's make the best of the opportunity that living with type 1 diabetes presents. Let's all work to develop and own those life skills that living with this condition gives us, helping us to grow as healthy, happy, and no-limits successful people! And I urge you to make the best out of this opportunity NOW. With all the ongoing work and research in the area of type 1 diabetes, this opportunity might not be there forever.

www.behavioraldiabetes.org (The Behavioral Diabetes Institute)

www.ayudainc.net (American Youth Understanding of Diabetes Abroad)

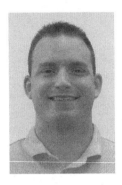

CHAPTER 14   *by Adam McLaughlin*

'Hello. My Name is Adam and I Have Diabetes'

Waking Up

"You can expect to be discharged within two weeks."

Those words from my nurse make up my first memory as a person with diabetes. She wasn't talking about my being discharged from the hospital—you see, at the time I was a Midshipman Third Class and a football player at the United States Naval Academy (USNA)—she was referring to my now-pending discharge from the Navy. No Caring. No Empathy. Nothing but those terrible words—and then she turned around and left.

So there I was, lying in a hospital bed at the National Naval Medical Center, dealing with my new reality as a person with diabetes and trying to figure out what I now wanted to do with my life. Before I knew it, a nurse stood in front of me with a needle full of insulin and asked me if she should stick me, or if I wanted to do it myself. I surprised even myself when I took it, and without a second thought, stuck the needle in my stomach. I don't remember if I did it right, or if it hurt, but that moment set the stage for what would eventually become my approach to this whole thing: I don't have a choice, so I just have to do it.

I thank God that I had such a solid support system over the next five days. Along with my mom, I had this wonderful new girlfriend, Rose, who didn't run away (and I should add that she is now my wife and soon to be the mother of my son!). While Rose was keeping my spirits as high as can be, my mother was keeping the hospital from sending me into insulin shock. Really! You're a nurse and you try to give me 20 units of fast-acting *Novolog* instead of long-lasting *Lantus*®??!! If my mother had not been there to catch it, the outcome would have been very bad.

The rest of my stay was pretty much a blur. I remember that my roommate was also a Midshipman, and also had just been diagnosed with diabetes, but he was a Junior and had already signed his papers, so he was able to stay in. I remember that we went out to the McDonalds® across the street and stocked the unit refrigerator full of cheeseburgers because the hospital thought that the best way to treat our diabetes was to starve us. I remember my Mom and Rose taking me to Fuddruckers® just down the street when I could get out for lunch. But most of all, I remember waking up every day dreading being released—because that meant that my all-too-short Naval career was that much closer to ending.

After I learned what was wrong with me, the previous months made sense to me. I had every single symptom on the posters: frequent urination, unquenchable thirst and hunger, weight loss, vision problems... the list goes on. But it was the last two that had me the most worried. For weeks I had had the thirst, hunger, and urination, and just put it in the back of my mind. However, the drastic weight loss and vision problems scared the heck out of me. I was a healthy twenty-one-year-old man in great shape, training not only to compete at the I-A level of college athletics, but also to serve in the Navy and one day to fly jets. Even with all the working out, lifting, eating, and supplements, I had lost twelve pounds in less than three days. I also had lost my perfect 20/20 vision. At first I couldn't read the clock on the wall or the blackboard any longer, and I was eventually asking the guy next to me in class to read it to me so that I could take notes. My vision deteriorated to absolute blurriness; I could not make out the face of the person standing in front of me. Those two things were enough for me to schedule an appointment to see the doctor, and the outcome of that visit is history. Thankfully, just a few days after I began the insulin regimen, most of those symptoms went away; my vision went back to normal, and I had no problem bulking back up. And thankfully, to this day, I continue to live a life free of complications.

At that point, nothing could have convinced me that diabetes could be a "blessing in disguise," but through my journey I did, in fact, come to accept that point of view.

Mom's Story – Growing Up With Diabetes

My journey with diabetes did not begin on that fateful day of January 31, 2004. My mother, Patricia, who has type 1 diabetes as well, also was diagnosed when she was an adult. I would like to dedicate this chapter to my mother. Without her courage, guidance, and support, this new life of mine would be very different. Thank you, Mom. Together we will *dia-beat-this!*

I don't remember her diagnosis, or much of how it impacted her life at the time, mainly because she just didn't complain about it—and that no doubt was the basis of my attitude towards my diabetes after I was diagnosed. I grew up watching her give herself shots, often asking her, "Mom, how do you do that?" and following it up with "I could never do that, Mom. You're so brave!"

It didn't really have much of an effect on me, again because she didn't let it. Of course, I knew when she had low blood sugar or when it was high, but not for many years did I truly understand what that really meant. I didn't understand why she needed that orange juice "right now" and why it couldn't wait until I finished the next level of my video game or until the next commercial of my television program began. I didn't understand why she would suddenly be so grumpy from a low blood sugar reaction, or feel so crappy after she miscalculated her dinner *bolus*, and her blood sugar would be high all night. But like everything else, she took it in stride.

Learning to Cope

From there it was no smooth ride. Although my doctor provided some relief when he decided to not let the Navy discharge me until the end of the semester, that relief was short-term, because there was no changing the fact that I was on the way out. I went into a pretty deep depression for a couple of months. I didn't get out of bed. I didn't go to class. I made excuses to get one sick pass after another—until one day I finally snapped out of it. I had some fantastic friends, teammates, and squad mates—far too many to name here—but it was my roommates who had a lot to do with my turnaround. Tanner Garrett and Jason Bowers put up with my negative attitude day after day and helped pull me out the other side. After that day, I decided that I was going to make this disease fit into my life—not change my life to fit this disease.

The general ignorance about type 1 diabetes shocked me. Because I grew up around it, I didn't realize how little most people knew. The worst example of that happened when the head trainer of the team told me that some people had asked him whether my diabetes was *contagious*. Because of the all-too-numerous experiences like that, I made it a point to always correct the ridiculous things people would say or assume, and I continue to be surprised to this day how much educating I do almost daily. It infuriates me when someone says how "shocked" he or she is to hear that I have diabetes—"after all, you're not old or fat."

Three months after my diagnosis, I had my first true trial—Spring Break in Mexico with the football team. Although my doctor wasn't very happy about it, and my mother, to say the least, didn't approve, the trip had already been paid for before my "new friend D" came into my life. And besides, it was literally my last hurrah with the boys! Thankfully, I had entered my *honeymoon phase* just prior to going, which made the management of my regimen much easier. From the beach all day to the clubs all night, I did what I had to do to keep myself safe while taking full advantage of our very short time away from the Academy. I tested constantly and brought my meter and insulin with me everywhere we went. Even with all the "partying" we did, and the awful carbohydrate-heavy Mexican food we endlessly enjoyed, I did not need a drop of insulin the entire trip.

I found that humor was a great way for me to deal with the odd looks or questions I would get. One night, an underclassman came into our room to talk to one of my roommates, and I just happened to have a needle in my butt giving myself my nightly *Lantus*® shot. He froze in horror (you have to remember that I was playing football, and I was quite a big guy then) and stammered through an excuse to leave, professing that he didn't see anything. Of course we couldn't let that one go and had to have a little fun with the kid for a while.

The End of My World as I Knew it

The next step on my journey was two-fold: Where would I go to school? And what would I do with my life? Due to my athletics, I wanted to transfer to a good I-AA school so that I could continue playing without sacrificing a year of eligibility, but I wasn't a star, by any means, so I had to do my own recruiting. I contacted a lot of schools that fit the criteria: some were open to talking, while others simply said to forget it because of the diabetes. In the end, I decided to attend Villanova University. Not only did they have a good football program with a solid reputation and a well known, successful coach, but they also had a superb business school. One of my lifelong friends, Sean Stevenson, had a very successful sales career, and since I had already all but flunked out of my Computer Science track at the USNA after trying to follow the path of my brother, Constantine, I figured business was my best bet.

After those decisions were made, the last weeks at the Academy turned out to be some of the toughest times of my life. I was beyond distraught that, after three years of being side-by-side, I was forced to abandon those whom I was supposed to go to war with. Saying goodbye to my friends and teammates, who felt more like my brothers and sisters, was not easy. I did not know if I would ever see some of those men and women again and, unfortunately, some were lost in defense of this great country. I'm not nearly vain enough to think that, if I were still in, I could have prevented any of it; but I will never be okay with the fact that I was not.

The support I had from those with whom I had become the closest got me through those last weeks. I doubt that he even remembers it, but one "brother" of mine, Dan Gibbon, said to me as I was on my way out of the gate for the last time, "I don't understand why the worst things happen to the best people." To this day, that was among the most impactful things anyone has ever said to me.

His words inspired me to be the best man I can possibly be. It made me want to make the most of this new life I was starting.

Transitioning to This New Life

Once I was out of the care of the Navy doctors, my first order of business was to find a new one. I was fortunate to find a doctor right away who worked with me and helped me in my goal to make this disease fit into my life (rather than one who would try to make me change in ways that would make this transition more difficult). I had lucked out, and my first real-world doctor was fantastic. He worked with me in every way I asked him to, and he made it clear that he shared my "make-it-work-for-you" attitude. In fact, to this day, the only dietary change I made was to stop drinking sugar, and that's only because I chose not to waste insulin on what I drank. However, he did not understand the requirements that my athletic life had on my diabetes, and I soon was searching for a doctor who did. That's when I had the good fortune to meet Gary Scheiner, MS, CDE, and Founder of Integrated Diabetes Services outside of Philadelphia. It was as if he understood every issue that I was going through, both on the field and in the classroom. After just my first meeting with him, I had a whole new insulin regimen with which to attack my workouts, and a new vision with which to attack my diabetes. My time with Gary was all too short: my insurance would not reimburse for his services, and I could not afford more than a couple of months while trying to pay my way through school. In my short time with Gary (and this is no exaggeration), he changed my life with diabetes.

Aside from adjusting to a new team and having to make all new friends, my transition to Villanova was relatively seamless. I have never been shy about anyone knowing I have diabetes, so I did not have any issues with any of my new friends, teammates, or classmates seeing me test my blood sugar. For the most part, my teachers either didn't mind or were helpful with my needs, but there were some who were just a pain. One whom I remember in particular either just didn't believe me or didn't care. It happened to be my first class of the morning, and one day my blood sugar was so dangerously low after a morning workout that I had to go eat something instead of coming to class. He didn't want to hear my reasons for missing his class, and he held against me, in my grade, any days that I missed due to diabetes issues.

One great surprise was that there was another man with diabetes on the team! Bryan Adams was a big help as I went through the trial and error process of figuring out my insulin dosing and food regimen so that I could make it through a practice or workout without wild swings in my blood sugar management. For the most part, the coaching staff and trainers at Villanova were much more accepting and supportive than what I had experienced during my last months at the Academy, which I'm sure was directly due to having had Bryan around for the previous two years.

Eventually I figured out what worked for me. An issue I did repeatedly have to deal with, however, was the ignorance of the student trainers. They often were clueless as to how to treat any issues that arose, especially a low blood sugar reaction. An all too frequent encounter went something like this: As we were warming up for a game, for some reason my blood sugar would drop. Not wanting to miss too many drills, I would discretely ask a student trainer for glucose tabs, and he would then hand me *two* tabs and tell me to come back in *thirty* minutes if I needed more. Under no circumstance would they give me any more than two tabs, repeatedly citing what they thought was the "guideline" for treating a low blood sugar. (Of course they didn't even know that they were wrong about that, too: Two tabs is only eight grams of carbohydrate, while the guidelines are to take fifteen grams of carbohydrate and wait fifteen minutes.) At that time, I was about 265 pounds, engaged in high-impact exercises, and had to argue with some student about treating my plunging low blood sugar… frustrating would be quite an understatement! Eventually, after I raised enough of a commotion, the head trainer would come over and hand me what I needed.

It was at Villanova that I found my passion, helping young athletes with diabetes, because I had seen first hand the discrimination that followed a diagnosis of diabetes, especially in athletics. I was asked to be a member of a panel at the annual meeting of the Diabetes Exercise and Sports Association (DESA). It was an extremely humbling yet inspiring experience: I was on a panel with professional athletes who had excelled at their respective sport in spite of having diabetes. (At that time, I had not yet competed since my diagnosis.) To this day, I do not know why they asked me to be on the panel, but I am certainly glad they did. To see and hear how successful those athletes were was extremely helpful to me as I began my climb back. I learned just how much fun it was to talk to the kids and their parents and to help them through their tough times.

Because of my work with DESA, I became acquainted with Dr. Matthew Kane, who ran a program for young athletes with diabetes. Once every couple of months, we would get together with the kids and their families and just have a great time. The main part of the program was to educate the kids and their parents and do our best to prepare them to be successful athletes, despite their diabetes. But, of course, we would have some fun while doing it, usually by playing some sort of game that gave the parents an idea of what it was like to have diabetes. Bryan even joined me for some meetings. That was the foundation for my passion and what I would eventually choose to do with my life and diabetes.

When my football career ended, I made what would prove to be the most pivotal change in my diabetes management: I finally went on an insulin pump. I had resisted it while I was playing because I just didn't want to have to worry about a site being banged around on the field and having to change it more frequently. I had no idea what a difference a pump would make for me compared to shots. No longer was I stuck on an insulin regimen. No longer did I have to take multiple shots to cover a single meal when I would eat a lot (which is frequently). Now I could control my insulin more precisely and make corrections that were more minute than I ever could with a syringe. But most importantly for me, I could now fine-tune my workouts.

Finally All Grown Up

Well, eventually the day came: After seven long years and two schools, I did actually graduate! I accepted a job with Becton Dickinson, which required a move from central Pennsylvania to Long Island, New York. A new life awaited me and my diabetes: I had to find multiple new doctors, a new pump trainer, and a new gym, and to start a new job. Basically, that was the scariest thing for me—a whole new daily routine. But I didn't have to do it all alone.

Rose, the love of my life, turned out to be the best "type 3" that anyone could ever have. ("Type 3" is what I call anyone who lives with a person with diabetes, because sometimes it runs their life too.) Somehow, I convinced her to quit her career, sell her house, and move to Long Island with me, and I'm still trying to figure out how I pulled that one off! From the little thoughtful things she did—like carrying bigger purses that fit all of my kits and supplies and just knowing when to get me the bottle of glucose tablets—she has been by my side literally from day one. Although, in moments of weakness, she will admit that her lack of understanding about the nuances of this disease are frustrating to her, she has been nothing but steadfast in her support. I could write an epic novel to rival Homer about how fantastic she is, and there still wouldn't be enough words to truly describe it. Honey, thank you for all that you do!

After a year of transition in New York, I decided to finally get involved again. Through my job, I got connected with Winthrop Hospital's Diabetes Education Department and became involved with their "Kindred Spirits" Support Group. This is a support group for families of children with diabetes, run by Eileen Eagan, FNP-C, CDE. Rose and I would play with the kids and help teach them about living life with diabetes. When needed, I would speak to the parents about how their kids can successfully be active and engage in athletics while controlling their diabetes.

Then, I found JDRF (formerly the Juvenile Diabetes Research Foundation International, but now just JDRF). Not having grown up with diabetes, I knew nothing about JDRF, but when it came up on an Internet search, I reached out to them for any support I could get. They say timing is everything, and in this instance it couldn't have been more true. I called the office on a Thursday, and they asked me to speak at their Educational Seminar that Saturday on the Athletes With Diabetes panel. It was there that I developed my opening line for my speeches. In keeping with my sense of humor, and using it to deal with diabetes, I would begin my talks in the likeness of an AA (Alcoholics Anonymous) meeting. I would say to them: "Hello. My name is Adam, and I have diabetes." And then they would respond with: "Hello, Adam. Welcome." After that experience, I was hooked, and now I do anything I can for them. Whether it's speaking at their numerous seminars, being a mentor to a kid with diabetes, helping out in the office, or anything else they need, I can't get enough of it. I was beyond honored when, two years ago, they asked me to join the Board of Directors for the Long Island chapter, then a year later, to take on a leadership role as the Treasurer. But as great as these two years have been, I'm really looking forward to the next two, because I have been asked to take on two new roles. The first is to serve as Outreach Chair, working with the most awesome person in the world—Betsy Paffmann, the Outreach Coordinator, who is the mother of a child with type 1 diabetes and who runs the best outreach program in the country! I've also been asked to serve as the Activation Coordinator for the Government Relations Advocacy Team.

That's All, Folks

Although it's not the life I had planned for myself, my life now is great. I have a wonderful family, a great job, fantastic friends… and a son on the way!! In fact, by the time you read this chapter, Jonathan Frank McLaughlin will officially be a part of our family. I still strive to stay in great shape, as Rose and I are amateur fitness buffs. We work out as frequently as we can and have even participated in a couple of Sprint-triathlons over the past two years. (My wife will be very upset if I don't say that she has beaten me every time!)

If I can leave you with some words of wisdom that I've learned the long and hard way about dealing with diabetes, they would be the following:

1. First and foremost, figure out how to make diabetes fit into your lifestyle, not change your lifestyle for diabetes.
2. Secure your support system and educate them on what you need and how they can best support you.
3. Find a doctor who will work with you and help you make diabetes fit into your lifestyle. If you don't feel that he or she does, then get a new one.
4. Get on a pump! I am a huge pump pusher—after fighting it for so long and then seeing what a difference it makes in my life everyday, I am a huge believer.
5. Help others. It has been so rewarding and helpful in managing my own diabetes to know that I have had an impact on others. If you're not already involved, call the JDRF and ask them what you can do for them. (For further information about JDRF, please see the website listed at the conclusion of this chapter.)

And that's my story. If there's even one person out there who is helped and inspired by my story, then it was worth putting down on paper. I wish you nothing but the best in your life; and there is absolutely nothing you can't do just because you have diabetes. Get out there and live life to the fullest. When it gets you down, or diabetes has you in a funk, just remember: IT'S ONLY DIABETES! If you take care of yourself and are diligent about your regimen, you will live a long and healthy life. With a little effort, you can make diabetes your own blessing in disguise.

www.jdrf.org (JDRF)

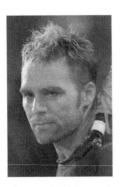

CHAPTER 15 *by Hamish Richardson*

Livin' the Dream

If there was no cloud cover at night, you could be assured that you'd wake to a white landscape—frost half an inch thick covering everything. Yes, the Bathurst winters, in New South Wales, were cold. We were three hours west of Sydney, Australia, over the Blue Mountains.

I'm sure that my mum's old ski gloves helped a bit, but by the time I had peddled the fifteen minutes uphill to school, my fingers would be frozen. So, too, my toes. So, too, the water fountains—"bubblers," as we call them.

Nothing, literally, would thaw until about eleven o'clock, when the sun inevitably and deliciously would break through the dense fog that accompanied every frost.

I remember this because I remember the excruciating thirst. By the end of that short bike ride, my eleven-year-old body would be screaming for water. In vain, I would twist the faucet on a bubbler—the clear plug of ice in the hole at the top serving only to torment me like the jibes of a playground bully.

Of course, once they came to know more, my parents realised that all of the symptoms probably had been there. Along with the unquenchable thirst, I was urinating like a racehorse; feeding like a ravenous shark; losing weight; listless... but back then, who knew? Particularly when a kid was keeping pace with siblings and friends.

They reckon that it must have gone on like that for weeks until good old Mother's instinct kicked in—that it wasn't just a passing phase or a growth spurt that her eldest child was going through. She took me to Dr. Pepper—yes, that's right, the real Dr. Pepper—our gentle, old family doctor.

Later that night, I was sitting up in the middle of my parent's double bed when the phone rang. My blood test results were back, and Dr. Pepper wanted me brought straight up to hospital. Mum and Dad delivered the news with a bowl of dessert.

Then the torture began. I wasn't allowed to eat anything for maybe a day and a half, and when food finally came, it made me feel sick trying to get anything down. There was the intravenous drip stuck into a vein on the top of my left hand, which ached more and more as the days went by, and that blood-testing regimen. I came to dread the appearance of the friendly pathologist. He wielded the professionals-only precursor to today's personal blood sugar meter. Not like today's spring-loaded pricking device with the smallest of points, his was a little piece of metal that came to an arrowhead. He'd firmly pinch the end of one of my fingers before effecting a quick, efficient, painful jab. He would do this a few times every day, and I remember him joking that he was running out of fingers... no joke to me. In the end, when I saw him coming, I would frantically begin scratching at the most recently pricked site, desperate to coax a drop of blood to the surface and avoid another painful puncturing, all the while trying to hold back the tears.

Of course it wasn't all bad. The nurses were caring, Dr. Pepper always lovely, my sister and two brothers visited, my friends came by... but after two weeks, I was simply bored out of my brain. Any novelty had long worn off, and the only highlight of each day was the arrival of the next meal. Maybe that's where I learnt to savour my food—because I knew there wouldn't be any seconds.

After three weeks, I felt like I was in prison.

Two things happened during my incarceration, which I suspect had a bearing on how I would approach a lot of things after that: the first was SNOW!

I awoke one morning with everyone abuzz. Although "below freezing" was typical for a Bathurst winter, our elevation was not high enough for any kind of regular snowfall. That morning, the world outside was as I'd never seen it. If the frosts were a thin sheet of ice, this was a soft, thick, enticing blanket of white. I imagined the fun everyone would be having at school and could hardly bear the thought that I was missing out.

I've never missed out again—on anything.

And then there was that orange.

The truth was, I'm told, that I had been at Death's door. Stabilising my blood sugar took time. Finally, some kind of balance had returned, and only one thing stood between me and freedom.

"As soon as you can give your own injection, you can go home," Dr. Pepper told me. The gauntlet had been thrown.

The nurses set me up with syringe and needles and an orange to practise on. (I kept that severely skewered citrus as a souvenir for much longer than I should have.) A few days later, with my family, Dr. Pepper, nurses, pathologists, and kitchen staff gathered around my bed, I took the plunge.

No one else has ever given me an insulin injection since.

Independence and determination: I think as much as anything, they're a state of mind.

Diabetes. It was a new word for all of us, and our family life would never be quite the same again.

Certainly much fell back into how it had been—picnics out to the river, imaginary adventures in the backyard, piano lessons, *The Wonderful World of Disney* on the black and white "telly" on a Sunday night that always signalled the end of another weekend.

It was the *detail* that brought about the shift, and over the years it was the element that, in moments of frustration, I resented most. From time to time, I have thought how much easier diabetes could have been handled if it had just been a case of shoot-up and forget; but that's not how it goes. With diabetes, the devil's in the details, and it was so much worse back then. The measuring out of the few teaspoons of butter that I was allowed each day, counting how many slices of toast I could have for breakfast, salad every lunch, or servings of vegetables that I had to have with dinner, skim milk—watery, tasteless... everything in measured portions. I couldn't have more even if I wanted it, and I needed to consume the daily requirement even if I didn't feel like it.

It was the mid-1970s, and the approach to diabetes management was... inflexible. It was also rudimentary compared to today's innovations.

Reusable "horse needles" and foaming test tubes: I have said this often when asked to recount what it was like being a child with diabetes. No ultra-fine needles or insulin pumps. The glass syringe and screw-on needle would be kept sterilised in "Metho"—methylated spirits—or boiled before my morning injection. I can remember sometimes sitting for half an hour trying to get that stubborn thing into my leg. I shudder at the thought now.

Back then, to get a rough indication of what your blood sugar was doing, you had a set-up like a school science lab. You'd urinate in a jar, then measure out and add things to test tubes before comparing resulting colours against a chart. If the "pee sticks" that came later—and did the same job without the mad scientist scenario—made life a bit easier, the development of personal blood sugar monitoring units was a revolution.

Looking back, my overall sense was that having diabetes never stopped me from doing or being anything I wanted. And that does hold true. I have given that reassurance to many newly diagnosed kids and their parents over the years. By the same token, certainly I had my moments.

I dealt with any newfound notoriety at school by refusing to feel embarrassed by the attention, as much as that was possible—made easier, perhaps, by the fact that I had already decided that I wanted to be a "pop star."

Clearly though, there was a bit of putting on a brave face, because it wasn't all smooth sailing.

There was the night of Icara McGovern's birthday party. Icara was my girlfriend. There with all my friends, newly diagnosed, not allowed to eat sweets, I knew I had one small window of opportunity. I rehearsed a plan in my head. As soon as the lights went out for the lighting of the cake, I sprang into action, reaching for the bowl of lollies in the middle of the table. Unfortunately, my timing was off, the lights came back on sooner than expected, and I was there like a kangaroo caught in a spotlight—leaning out across the table, arm extended to the forbidden fruit. Foiled, for the rest of the evening I contented myself by indulging in the only party food that was "free" for me—frankfurts. Those evil mini hot dogs, party franks, did taste pretty good. But too much of a good thing… my belly began to bubble in the middle of the pass-the-parcel game, and for the remainder of the gathering, it was all I could do to contain myself. The contents of my stomach were stewing like the magma of Mount Vesuvius. Arriving home at the end of the evening, I burst through the front door, bolted upstairs to the bathroom, and exploded.

To add insult to injury, I got to school the following Monday only to learn that Icara no longer wanted to be my girlfriend. My prepubescent heart was broken. Apparently I had been rude to her mum at the party—and deep down I suppose there may have been some truth to her accusations. I reckon it's likely that I was being a bit of a "smart-arse"—a little unconscious over-compensation going on. A young fella trying a tad too hard to fit back into a world that hadn't changed, while for him, everything had.

I'd like to be able to report that years later, as matured young adults, Icara and I met up, made amends, laughed about who we had been, and enjoyed a night together that neither of us would ever forget… But alas, none of that happened.

Growing up, I was a sportsman, a musician, a teenager... I was also a young person with diabetes. Now I am also a person who plays sport and makes music, a person in his late 40s and with children. The point is, I am who I am, I do what I do, I've got what I've got. No one thing defines me; I'm bits and pieces of a lot of things. And sometimes, things do define us, and that's okay. Later on, I did become a "pop star" in my own way. Touring for fifteen years with the independent world music band "BROTHER," there were thousands of fans for whom I was a musician. That's how they knew me, and that's how they saw me. And that was cool with me. But every night that I took to the stage, all of those CDs I signed, all of those dressing-room parties and late-night hotel-room gatherings, I still had diabetes. I was a person with diabetes, yes, but that one thing would never define me.

During my touring years in the U.S., I did quite a bit of work with *Children with Diabetes* and was a sometime "poster boy" for a big diabetes medical supplies company. There have been times, getting up in front of a bunch of conference-goers or kids with diabetes, that I have winced at the bestowed title of "role model." After all, I had been by no means a perfect patient of the pancreas. (Nobody is "perfect.") What I've come to appreciate is that it's all about balance.

Yes, you've got to be realistic—but you've also got to keep it real.

Through my high school years, I did every sport on offer—made the school swimming team, athletics team, tennis team, cross-country team. Occasionally, I stood out; usually, I was just pretty good. I was Pipe Major of the school bagpipe band when we won the Australian Junior Championships; learnt piano, clarinet, and guitar; had an ever-evolving rock band; and played in whatever musical was happening. The thing was, I wanted to do all that stuff. I suspect I would have been like that, diabetes or not. Then again, maybe I did have something to prove—at least to myself.

It still gets back to that simple philosophy: diabetes doesn't have to stop you from doing whatever you want to do. Attitude is everything. Logistics can always be worked out.

Sure, there have been times when I've wished that I didn't have diabetes—of course. But the "why-me?" wonderings don't get you very far, no matter who you are, unless you come to a positive conclusion. I wish to state for the record that, to date, there has been no big epiphany for me.

During my teenage years, any spare time on weekends and during the holidays would see the kids helping our parents on the farm—doing the cattle, fencing, watering trees through the drought, feeding out to the stock from the back of the ute, and keeping up with our enormous garden. Every summer, we'd have a couple of weeks at the beach. We were mad body surfers—pretty crazy, looking back—but we loved it. I loved it. I also loved rugby. I lived for the game they play in heaven, and went on to play four years of first grade at university while completing a journalism degree.

I think now of what it was like for me as a teenager with diabetes: infrequent testing, once-daily shots in the morning, scanning the dining hall tables at lunchtime for leftover slices of bread because I was still hungry, downing chocolate after school in anticipation of sports training with no idea whether I needed the sugar boost or not. I shake my head in disbelief.

Despite the knowledge with which we can approach things these days, I suspect that nothing has changed much for young people, who, of course, will always be teenagers first. Thank goodness that our bodies are very forgiving while we're young and still growing, and fit and active.

Management-wise, it wasn't much better at university. I'd sugar up before training or a rugby match and automatically have more glucose at half time—never twigging to the reason why I couldn't down a beer straight after the match like most of the blokes, but had to guzzle water. And then there was the whole social scene. I never went off the rails, but I had my moments of excess and indulgence.

The thing that worked in my favour, I reckon, was that I was incredibly fit, physically active almost every day, and, while I regularly may have given my diabetes the cold shoulder, I never forgot it was with me. Over the years, what has continued to stand me in good stead is thinking a bit ahead and taking a moment to check in on my diabetes. Really, it's always the times when I haven't done those things that I've been caught out. It's horrible being caught with no insulin, horrible being caught with no sugar, horrible recovering from a bad *hypoglycemic reaction*.

That's my advice these days: think ahead and check in. Do that, and diabetes won't rule your life. It's the old "stitch-in-time" philosophy.

With the way our brains are wired, we humans may simply be unable to fully comprehend the potential adverse ramifications of unchecked climate change—too big, too distant—but not so, unchecked diabetes management. Many of those associated ramifications play out pretty quickly and run the gamut of negatives: lack of energy, tight and uncomfortable muscles, thirst, crankiness, loss of focus, and even unconsciousness. And who needs any of that getting in the way of getting on with life? Thinking ahead, checking in—that puts you in control.

Not too long after I had started at university, I met with my new diabetes specialist in Sydney. Along with study, rugby, and a healthy social life (or perhaps that should be rugby, a healthy social life, and study?), I was performing with my brother a couple of nights a week in local pubs and clubs. Long, late nights messed not only with my sleep patterns, but inevitably with the diabetes also. Frustrated that his efforts to steer me to tighter control weren't being followed, the doctor put the question to me, "Can't you just have a normal job?"

But I had never tried to make my lifestyle fit my diabetes. With the support of my parents, it had always been about working out how my diabetes would fit my lifestyle. In those early years, there was a seemingly endless list of things you couldn't do. Literally, you shouldn't do these things—wear synthetic soled shoes, walk barefooted on the beach, scuba dive, sky jump, drink beer, play late-night gigs. Okay, so I took the advice and have never gone scuba diving. Never *yet*.

If we don't want to do something, we can always find an excuse. By the same token, we can always find a reason why we should try something. I hit the road with my brothers after finishing at university. Forging our own distinct sound, and as one of the first independent acts to eschew the big record labels, with BROTHER I recorded twelve albums; toured with Joe Walsh, Jon Entwhistle, Jeff "Skunk" Baxter, Keith Emmerson…. We played the Rock 'n' Roll Hall of Fame with Lincoln Park and Alecia Keys; wound up on the soundtracks for *Baraka* and *Twilight Zone*; had a cameo performance on *ER*; played all over the United States, Canada, France, and Egypt. (For further information about BROTHER, please see the website at the conclusion of this chapter.)

Along the way, I married my almost childhood sweetheart and was further blessed with two delightful daughters. They hit the road with the band, saw the world, and got a taste for music and travel before I headed home to grow veggies, body surf, and pick up the journalism thing.

You'll always be able to find elements of someone else's life that you wish you had—and there are some things that you can change if you really want or need to. Other things you have to accept. If it was announced tomorrow that they'd found a cure for diabetes, I would be delighted—and here's hoping. But I'd rather have diabetes than some of the life challenges that many others have to overcome. With diabetes, you can live an "ordinary" life—add extra spice to taste.

And, yeah, you do have to watch what you eat and when you eat it. You do have to press pause every now and again in order to check in. You do have to try to maintain a healthy diet and stay fit… what a drag.

It's almost forty years for me and diabetes; that's most of my life. And apart from the last couple of years, where I've had to have a few laser treatments on my eyes for some retinopathy, so far so good. I've had good periods of control and bad, good days and bad. Just got to keep learning, keep adjusting.

I miss playing rugby and those magic moments on stage with a great band. But I have loved being at home with no departure date looming, being able to massage my girls' feet every night as they fall off to sleep, being able to walk through the bush to the beach every day, and being involved in the life of a small, connected community. Some things come and go—others are with you for the duration. Either way, there's always something new to tackle. Recently, with three mates, I hiked the main range at Kosciusko in the Snowy Mountains, and with my sixteen-year-old elder daughter, have just qualified as a surf lifesaver.

I've been up and I've been down. Somewhere in it all there is balance.

I give thanks—life really is sweet.

As one fan in Paris kept shouting at me one night—"Livin' the dream, Brother—livin' the dream."

www.brothermusic.com

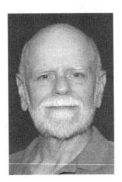

Photo credit by Leo Mahoney, Station Manager for CTSB- TV

CHAPTER 16   *by Will Ryan*

The 'Joyful Diabetic's' Journey

In the Beginning

I was very tired as I entered the high school locker room after a hard workout with the track team. I heard a commotion, but at first I couldn't see anything unusual because the lights were low. Then I noticed several older players huddled around Mike, a senior, who was lying on the floor. The coach was trying to revive Mike by pouring orange juice into his mouth. How, I wondered, could juice revive him? Five minutes later, Mike was awake and sitting up. The coach offered him a chocolate bar. Later I learned that Mike had passed out from diabetes. I figured that if the treatment for this disease was candy, it couldn't be that bad.

I can say with certainty that I didn't think about diabetes again until twenty-three years later. I was living in New Jersey and working in New York. Most mornings, I took the bus into Manhattan; however, it was becoming increasingly difficult to control my need to visit the men's room. I had an immense thirst and couldn't put the fire out. So, I stopped using the bus since it didn't have facilities, and I began driving to a parking lot in New Jersey for the Path train to the City. I could handle the thirty-minute drive, and then I used the station's restroom before boarding the train.

This was annoying, and I began talking about it with others. A nurse who lived across the street said, "I'll bet you have diabetes." I thought back to the locker room scene and began to worry about passing out. I was thirty-nine years old at the time and didn't have my own doctor, so I went to my son's pediatrician. He took a large drop of my blood and then told me to take a seat in his waiting room.

When I noticed the waiting room was full of mothers and children, I started to feel uncomfortable. I realized that I'd gone to the wrong type of doctor. In a few minutes, the doctor's head appeared through a partially opened door. He looked around and then made eye contact with me. In a loud voice, he called out, "You've got diabetes!"

I was stunned, shocked, and deeply embarrassed by this revelation. I wanted a hole to open in the floor and suck me in. I sheepishly left his office vowing never to return. He had wounded me, and I was hurt and angry. I went into denial. For the next year, I ignored my diabetes, hoping that the doctor was wrong and that my diabetes would go away. Of course, it's still with me after more than thirty-three years.

Waking Up to Diabetes

A year later, unrelated to my diabetes diagnosis, I separated from my family and moved to New York City to start a new life. I was referred to a consulting physician, Dr. Brown, an outstanding doctor who also taught medicine at Columbia Presbyterian Hospital. That's when I started taking care of my diabetes.

Under Dr. Brown's prescription and care, I began taking Diabenese®, got a blood glucose meter, and began testing my blood glucose on a regular basis. After an examination about a year later (I was then forty-one years old), he looked at my chart and then at me. "You may make it to age fifty... but you might not have your legs or your eyesight," he said. I was shocked and started to ask him what to do, but he interrupted me. "You've got to lose weight," he said. I weighed nearly 230 pounds on a five-foot-nine-inch body—way too much weight for my height. Next, I asked him how much I should weigh. I'll never forget what he said. I expected him to give me a number based on my height and body type; however, he said something quite different. "When you stand naked in front of a full length mirror and like what you see, you're there." Wow, what a great concept. That led to a serious weight-loss campaign. However, I must say, I've never been comfortable looking at my naked body, particularly now that gravity has had seventy-plus years to push my weight south.

Caring for Myself

I began my weight-loss campaign by joining the NY Road Runners Club. I enjoyed the camaraderie of the group and benefitted from instruction on how to run efficiently. I'm not one for moderation. I often say that I have an on/off switch without a rheostat. I ran nearly every day and competed in more than twenty 10K races in one year. My switch was on.

Between 1981 and 1983, I was in the best shape of my adult years. I lost about sixty pounds and felt wonderful. I even ran a half marathon, for which my goal was to average eight-minute miles for the 13.1 miles of the race. Since I wasn't a distance runner in high school or college, this was a challenge. There was a large clock with the running time available at every mile. At the first mile, my split was 7:15, and I worried about whether I could finish the event. I consciously slowed down; however, at the second split, my time was 14:20, which meant that I had actually sped up. I wasn't really worried since I felt super. When I completed the run, my average time was just under 7:30 per mile. I was amazed at my accomplishment.

My running partner, Elizabeth, was a much younger woman who was very strong and, thus, a challenging running partner. I fell in love with her, and we were married a year later. Elizabeth and I ran together frequently, including across the Golden Gate Bridge in San Francisco while on our honeymoon.

In those early days of caring for my diabetes, I learned a valuable lesson. Since I'm responsible for managing my blood sugar all the time, "It's up to me" became my mantra. Over time, I've become grateful for my diabetes. I've learned so much about how my body works and how things in my life impact my blood sugar level: exercise, food, worry, stress, and much more.

Transformation

I was doing well professionally. I was Vice President of Systems for Columbia Records—in those days part of CBS. Later, I was recruited to be Senior Vice President of Systems for the Travel Division of American Express®.

On my own time, I was taking a different path. I began a spiritual quest to understand the world of consciousness. I was inspired by *Out on a Limb* by Shirley MacLaine. Fascinated by her spiritual quest, I decided to take a journey of my own. I had many spiritual teachers and among them was Reiki Master, Michelle Trois. She was an opera singer who learned the Reiki energy transfer process to treat her vocal cords so that constant use would not negatively impact her singing. I, too, became a Reiki master and, in addition to healing my body and treating my diabetes, I was privileged to join a group of Reiki practitioners who treated people at the United Nations. Employees were from many countries, and nearly all were under stress. We were able to relieve some of their stress by giving them Reiki treatments during their lunch breaks. This experience taught me how much I enjoyed helping others.

William Sloan Coffin, the Senior Minister at Riverside Church in New York City, was a major influence on my life during those years. Bill became my friend and mentor. Having been the Chaplain at Yale University, as well as a Freedom Rider with Martin Luther King, Jr., he was a perfect leader for me to follow as I learned more about my own spirituality.

My evenings and weekends were spent with healers and people who were devoted to helping others. My days in the corporate world were a sharp contrast. So, in 1987, I quit my six-figure job and started working at a crystal shop in Greenwich Village. My corporate friends were shocked. How could I transform into a minimum-wage worker overnight? But, I found it was perfect for me during my transformative period. I wore jeans to work, listened to wonderful New Age music, and hung out with people healing themselves with crystals. Although I loved this portion of my life, I knew it was temporary. I had become calm as I basked in the positive energy of crystals.

Of course, these changes had a dramatic, positive impact on managing my blood sugar. My view of diabetes was also transitioning from a curse to a blessing. After four months at the store, I left to start my first consulting company, The Personal Development Corporation.

During the nearly ten years that I lived in New York City, I also went through a major transformation in my health. Although I was not seeing an endocrinologist, my consulting physician, Dr. Brown, was monitoring my type 2 diabetes. During this period, I started using a blood glucose meter, and I created a spread sheet to track my blood sugar levels. I used the tabular information to create a graph of my blood glucose. I called it the Graphic Control System. Here's how it worked: If I was considering eating a high-carbohydrate food like chocolate layer cake (my favorite), I would visualize my control graph. I imagined the large, high blood glucose spike in the graph that the cake would cause. Since I didn't want that, I skipped the cake. By just visualizing the graphic impact, I was able to reject the sugar-raising food.

A Move to the Country

Toward the end of my time in New York, my mother and sister were considering a change of their own, and they enrolled me in their project. They wanted to own and run a country inn. My young wife, Elizabeth, had gone her own way, so I joined them. The search, which began in Bucks County Pennsylvania, ended in the Berkshire Hills of Western Massachusetts. Right in the middle of the hectic 1990 summer season, the Ryan family took possession of the Williamsville Inn in West Stockbridge, MA.

That fall, I attended a mini reunion for Brown University's class of 1962. There I met and fell in love with my classmate, Susanna. We had not known each other at college. Six weeks later we were living together in Lee, MA, and the following September, we married on the lawn of the family inn.

Over the years I've found that a loving and supportive partner makes sugar management easier. My first wife resented me and my diabetes. Elizabeth was very compassionate and supported me without learning much about diabetes. Susanna, the love of my life, is a partner with me in dealing with my diabetes. She has researched and studied diabetes and participates in my major decisions, such as going on insulin, which I did in 1992.

It wasn't until I started using insulin, thirteen years after being diagnosed, that I became really serious about blood sugar management. Now we had an added concern—taking too much insulin and having a low blood sugar reaction. I remember experiencing a low blood sugar reaction right after I started taking insulin. I had tunnel vision along with sweating and reduced cognitive function. As I peered out of the fog from my low blood sugar, my brain kicked in telling me that I needed to *do* something. Instinctively, I reached for my insulin, but then a blaring voice went off in my head saying, *"No!"* This experience taught me about the dangers of having low blood sugar. I also learned that I needed to test more frequently—six to eight times per day since my blood sugar readings were the only way to use insulin properly and achieve self-care mastery.

I made some classic mistakes in my early weeks of injecting insulin. This one stands out in my memory. I was in Chicago for a business meeting, and several of us decided to take a taxi to a restaurant we had chosen. I knew that taking insulin in a restaurant would be challenging, so I tested my blood sugar and injected insulin while in my hotel room. I had forgotten about the time to get to the restaurant, and we got into serious traffic. I sensed that my sugar was very low, since my vision was blurred and I was sweating. Joe, the guy sitting next to me in the taxi, also had type 2 diabetes, and he knew the symptoms of low blood sugar. When the cab stopped, Joe ran into the restaurant and returned promptly with two dinner rolls, which I ate immediately. In fifteen minutes or so, my blood sugar was probably in the normal range, but again another mistake: I didn't have my blood glucose meter with me. I learned from this experience to never inject until food is in sight and to always have my meter with me.

I used to test and inject insulin at the table in restaurants; however, I noticed that some people were squeamish about seeing me do this, so I started testing in the men's room. One day, the restaurant manager came barging into the restroom loudly saying, "A guest reported to me that someone was doing drugs in here. Are you doing drugs?" Since I had just given myself an injection, the insulin and associated materials were on the counter. I replied, "Yes. I've just given myself a shot of insulin." His face turned crimson as he apologized and left the room. The lesson for me was to return to testing and injecting at the table. Diabetes is much more prevalent these days, and most people are used to seeing those with diabetes treat themselves in public places.

Lifestyle Changes

By this time, I was no longer involved with the inn and had started my own consulting business that combined my two passions—sales and computers. The Systems Sales Support Company provided consulting and product training to international companies around the world. My schedule, which was not of my own making, could have me teaching one class in Houston on a Friday and another in Singapore early the following week. Being on insulin required the additional burden of carefully packing the medication to keep it fresh, carrying enough testing strips to handle any unforeseen contingencies, and dealing with crossing many time zones that added to the challenge of eating on a schedule. I learned that my system did not react well to the stress of travel. In spite of setbacks, such as high blood sugar, I kept at it and eventually developed a routine that worked.

During those years, my endocrinologist, Dr. James Desemone, kept encouraging me to go on an insulin pump. As a type 1 pump user himself, he assured me that it would make blood sugar management much easier, especially since my lifestyle included business travel. But I was resistant. I was reluctant to have something attached to my body 24/7. How would I sleep?

Eventually I decided to start using an insulin pump, and I'm delighted with that decision, since it has helped me achieve an A1c of less than 7% for more than a decade. When I started using the insulin pump, Dr. Desemone told me to, "Think like a pancreas." Over the years, that advice has stayed with me. It helped me stay in touch with my body and its needs, which is an important source of joy with diabetes.

I had to stop running because of a painful hip, but moving to the country provided a much better environment for bicycling, one of my favorite exercises. A friend and cycling buddy suggested that we enroll in a 150-mile diabetes ride from Boston to Provincetown. More miles than I had ever cycled before, the event loomed as an enormous challenge. As the big day approached, I prepared for the ride by taking many longer practice runs around the hilly Berkshires. One of my concerns was how much insulin to take during the very long first leg from Boston to Hyannis, MA, a distance of one hundred miles. I packed plenty of diabetes supplies and food to eat. Along the way, the organizers provided food and water. Since it was a diabetes ride, the food was healthy, such as bananas and granola bars. At each break, I tested and, much to my surprise, I took no insulin while riding during the two-day event. I was burning calories at a high rate and my body was using all the sugar in my system, since muscles take what they need from the blood stream without needing insulin. That experience demonstrated the great value of exercise.

Although I haven't done another major ride like that since, I exercise almost every day. When I'm not cycling or snowshoeing, I walk. I wear a pedometer on the other side of my body from my pump, and many days I achieve my goal of 10,000 steps. The exercise improves my overall health and well-being and helps me keep my weight in range. Thank goodness, I never gained back the sixty pounds that I lost in the early days of my diabetes.

My Medical Team

As I began to embrace my diabetes and take more responsibility for managing my relationship with it, I realized that I needed a medical team to work with me. I told my endocrinologist, Dr. Desemone, that I saw him and the rest of the medical team as my coaches. I listen to them, but I'm in charge of my diabetes. Dr. Desemone liked my attitude on diabetes ownership and agreed with my approach.

I added an ophthalmologist, Dr. Shouldice, to look after my eyesight. It was he who operated on my cataracts a few years later, and now I've got my pilot's vision back. (I was a private pilot in my early thirties.) My ear doctor, Dr. Cavalli, was added when my hearing was waning. Ultimately, he recommended hearing aids. It took me a while to get used to them, but now I think they're wonderful. Dr. Greene is my dermatologist, and he's responsible for coaching me regarding ring worm and athletes foot. I'm susceptible to diabetes-related skin conditions, and he's a valued member of my team.

The team idea goes both ways. I learned that I can be helpful to medical practitioners as well. Dr. Eric Bush, my primary care physician, told me that he has learned more about diabetes from me than he had in medical school twenty-five years earlier. And since my doctors are my coaches, I make changes from time to time. After reading an article in a diabetes publication about what podiatrists should be checking for in people with diabetes, I sought a new foot doctor.

About five years ago, Dr. Desemone's practice changed, which meant that I had to find a new endocrinologist. I tried several endocrinologists over the next two years and finally went back to Dr. Jill Abelseth at The Endocrine Group in Albany, NY. She had been my doctor a few years back, and I was impressed with her, but the practice seemed like a diabetes factory. I'm still not pleased with the size of the group, but my visits with her are pure joy. We've even partnered on several webinars sponsored by Medtronic.

Most recently, I've added a cardiologist, Dr. Lisa Massie. She joined my team because I was experiencing erratic heartbeats. After many tests, including a stress test using a nuclear material, she suspected that I had blockage in the blood vessels of my heart and ordered a cardiac catheterization to evaluate my condition. My surgeon for this procedure was Dr. Peterman, who practices at Baystate Medical Center in Springfield, MA. I was awake for the catheterization and watched on the monitor as the probe entered my heart. He injected a fluid that enabled us to see my heart blood vessels. In short order, he said, "There's the blockage. Your main heart artery is totally blocked!" A minute or so later, he exclaimed, "Wow, look at that. Your heart healed itself by developing new vessels that took up the load previously handled by the main artery. One of them is actually back-feeding to the other side of the blockage. You're one of the lucky ones who've had a natural by-pass." In a subsequent meeting with

Dr. Peterman, he said that being in good shape was the reason my body healed itself. I was thrilled and grateful for all those years of running, walking, cycling and hiking—they paid dividends.

Becoming the "Joyful Diabetic®"

Back in my New York City days, I joined Toastmasters International. Toastmasters is about public speaking and leadership. I helped to found a new club in New York City, in the mid-1980s, and took Susanna to a meeting of that group on our first date. As my overseas consulting began to taper off, I considered taking a leadership role in the Regional Toastmasters organization. After a year of consideration (and discussion with Susanna), I decided to take on a three-year leadership commitment to the organization.

In 2008, I decided to be a speaker/facilitator for gatherings of people with diabetes. I called myself the "Joyful Diabetic®" which intrigues my audiences and encourages them to pay attention to my message. I've spoken to dozens of groups in an effort to help them take responsibility for their diabetes and to facilitate a process that encourages audience members to have confidence in their ability to manage their blood sugar. I normally work with a Certified Diabetes Educator and, for many events, my partner was Connie Hanham-Cain, RN, CDE. She's a great speaker and has a down-to-earth manner that enables people to get the message on how to manage blood sugar. I focus on the non-medical topics like diabetes ownership, responsibility, and commitment, while Connie handles the medical aspects of diabetes care.

Most of my audiences ask me how I can be joyful while "suffering" with diabetes. I tell them that, initially, I managed my blood sugar—while at the same time, hating my diabetes—with an inner dialogue saying, *"Why me?"* and *"It's not fair!"* I then go on to explain that negative thinking makes blood sugar management MUCH more difficult. Being joyful is a choice that any of us can make, and this decision is essential to achieving mastery.

I was invited to be the final speaker at the Diabetes Boot Camp for adults at the Hungerford Diabetes Center in Torrington, CT. At dinner, before I spoke, the conversation was about living with diabetes. I mentioned the importance of frequent blood sugar testing. The woman sitting next to me said, "I don't test." After taking this in, I asked her why. She said, "If my blood sugar is high, it will ruin my day." I agreed that I'd had the same thought, and then I asked her about the risks of not knowing if her blood sugar was low. We had an interesting conversation at the table and came to the consensus that high blood sugar takes much longer to kill you and that low blood sugar, if not treated quickly, can produce unconsciousness and ultimately death. We collectively made the point that, as they say on the diabetes cable television show, *dLife*: "Test! Don't guess." At the end of my session, one of the leaders told me that the woman had declared that she was committed to testing at least four times per day.

It's situations like this that inspire both my public speaking and my blog writing. I began blogging in November, 2008 and, by the summer of 2012, had posted over 160 entries. (For further information about my motivational speaking engagements and my blog, please see the website at the conclusion of this chapter.)

Managing Emotions

Over my diabetes years, I've noticed that strong emotions create chaos with my blood sugar. For example, anger causes my body to release adrenalin in case I want to fight or run. Of course, this is a biological carry-over from early human existence. When anger kicks in, my adrenal glands secrete adrenalin into my blood stream, and this in turn causes my liver to release glucose to support the "fight or flight" reaction. This action directly increases my blood sugar—not a good thing for those of us with diabetes. Since we can't alter the body's normal function, the only option is to control emotions. Of course, this is much easier said than done. On the other hand, I've found a process that works.

When I sense anger, I pay attention to what I'm thinking. I typically discover that I'm thinking negative thoughts, which are causing the anger. Since I'm in charge of my thinking, most of the time, I'm able to start thinking about my grandchildren—always a source of joy. In no time, the anger goes away and along with it a cessation of adrenalin release. I've found that this process really works and has helped me control blood sugar highs.

Lessons Learned

As I look back on my diabetes journey, here are some things I've learned:
- We cannot achieve diabetes mastery without taking ownership and responsibility.
- The single most important element in blood sugar management is attitude.
- Henry Ford was right when he said, "If you think you can do a thing or think you can't do a thing, you're right." A positive mental outlook is critically important to achieving self-care mastery.
- Since our muscles absorb glucose from our blood stream without insulin, all forms of exercise reduce our blood sugar level—even walking!
- My doctors are my coaches.

I am committed to personal growth, and diabetes has offered me many opportunities.

Achieving self-care mastery is difficult and has taught me that perfection is a direction rather than a goal.

Acknowledgment: I'd like to thank my wife, Susanna Opper, for her skilled professional editing of this chapter. As in all things in my life, her support is the wind beneath my wings.

www.JoyfulDiabetic.com

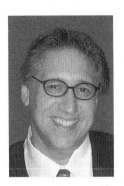

Photo credit by Marla E. Bayles

CHAPTER 17   *by Mitchell L. Schare, PhD, ABPP*

Poof – 522 and You're Type 2

"Poof – 522 and you're type 2." This quote is a bit of a lie; it's more of a paraphrase that represents the essence of what I heard and then felt at that moment. When my physician told me that my blood glucose level was 522 mg/dL, I sat there a bit stunned, pondering the number. I had no point of reference, so what did this mean? It didn't seem to be a good thing, because he quickly followed the revelation of the number with the announcement that I had diabetes. Huh? What? Just like that, a snap of the finger. Poof! Like a magician doing card tricks, here one moment, gone the next, first you don't have diabetes and then you do? At the age of forty-eight, it took just one pinprick of blood, and I was given this stigmatizing label and serious diagnosis. I was now a person with diabetes. My life as I had known it was gone, or so it seemed at that time.

My recall of what occurred that day in the Spring of 2005 is now a mixture of reality, emotion, and memory decay. In fact, the doctor was very gentle, supportive, and helpful as he spoke to me. I sat quietly, trying to absorb his explanation that a normal blood glucose reading for most people was between 90 mg/dL and 110 mg/dL. Needless to say a 522 mg/dL reading sounded scary, and from his serious tone, I knew that it was bad. He talked about food, gave me some basic dietary guidelines, and set up an appointment to see a diabetes educator. After getting medication instructions and some prescriptions, I found myself in my car driving home, feeling very alone, scared, and sad. Tears welled up in my eyes.

Denial and Avoidance

Denial and avoidance are problematic behaviors that most people engage in at some time in their lives. Denial and avoidance are concepts that I have studied for years; I am very familiar with them. As a Ph.D. in Clinical Psychology, I have spent many years developing areas of specialization that deal with these concepts. For example, I study the development and treatment of serious phobia, a manifestation of extreme anxiety. Phobic patients engage in avoidance of feared objects, situations, people, or places. This phobic avoidance causes sufferers to be unable to follow through on needed life activities, even putting important family and occupational obligations second to their fear. For example, aviophobic (fear of flying) patients will avoid flying to siblings' weddings, business meetings, parent's funerals, vacations, and many other life events. This avoidance can cause permanent fractures in families, loss of jobs, and dissolutions of marriages. Avoidance of something fearful and anxiety-provoking is a normal human reaction that most of us experience at times; however, too much avoidance is unhealthy behavior and typically warrants professional intervention.

Denial is a major concept that clinicians must overcome in working with patients who have alcohol and/or chemical dependencies. In my professional life, I have studied and treated numerous patients for problems of substance abuse, understanding the complex addictive nature of drugs and how they become intertwined in daily life. I strongly believe that, for many drug dependencies, such as alcohol or nicotine (typically via cigarettes), effective and conclusive methods to treat these problems exist. However, getting people to take advantage of these treatments can be a problem. Denial is the major handicap that we must learn to overcome. Drug abusers live in a world of denial. If people won't recognize (that is, they actively deny) that they have a problem, then they can convince themselves that they actually don't have one. Denial allows addicts' worlds to crumble around them as they begin to fail in their jobs, their family lives, and ultimately their health, without taking any responsibility for these events. The need for the drug is so strong that the abuser will just deny that need to avoid dealing with the potential loss of the substance. The best treatments for substance abuse can do nothing for an addict who won't engage in therapy due to their denial.

So now I will come clean with you. As I drove home that Spring day from my doctor's office, I realized that I was not only an expert who was knowledgeable about denial and avoidance, but I was an expert in living my own life of denial and avoidance! My physician really hadn't told me anything that I didn't expect to hear. Denial and avoidance are that powerful. I had successfully deceived myself for some time. I had successfully told myself that

I didn't have any problems. "I don't have to go to the physician for an exam; there is nothing wrong with me." I began to cry hard, as if I were mourning the life that I would never have again.

"Denying" Diabetes in My Family

During my late teenage years, my father had been diagnosed with type 2 diabetes when he was about fifty years old. Since I was off at college, I didn't hear much about this, except that he was being monitored well by his physician and all seemed in control. Perhaps this lack of inquiry on my part was due to my naiveté about diabetes, or my self-indulgent immersion into college life, but dad's problem was not discussed in phone calls or in person during breaks between semesters.

A few years later, while I was engaged in graduate studies, my sister Jane, four years my elder, had developed an unusual manifestation of type 1 diabetes. It was "unusual" to me in that she was diagnosed with Juvenile Diabetes at the age of twenty-eight. Jane had had a bad case of the flu, and within a few months she began to experience intense thirst. Shortly thereafter she was diagnosed and immediately became insulin-dependent. At a distance, I was sympathetic and concerned, but her problem seemed to be well under control. Years later, I learned that she was actually scared and depressed by her diabetes. My family has always been great and supportive of me, particularly in my educational endeavors. In retrospect, I now understand how much I was shielded from their individual difficulties as they arose. The only time I recall my sister's diabetes becoming a serious issue was during her pregnancy with twin girls. Her condition required very close monitoring and limited movement. It's easy to deny others' difficulties when they are not around you daily.

A Weighty Contribution

In general, my health has been good, except that I always had some tendency towards being overweight. It's very hard to simply analyze this issue. Some people like to thrust their hands out palms up and shout, "It's my genetics, and there is nothing I can do about this!" There may be truth, denial, or both operating in their thinking. Others learn food consumption patterns; that is when, what, and how to eat by emulating healthy and unhealthy family eating habits. Rather than be philosophical on this nature-versus-nurture inquiry, I'll just admit to being a combination of the two. I don't blame anybody; I just accept that weight issues have been part of my family's life.

Let me add that I like food. Quite a loaded statement, yet I have indeed met people who don't care for variety, spice, or adventure in their eating, qualities that I actively enjoy. There are people in the world who just eat until they have satisfied their hunger. I was the opposite of those people. When I was younger, more food was better, especially if it was starchy, carbohydrate-laden bread, rice, potatoes, and the like. I could easily consume a whole loaf of *challah* bread during a single snacking with just some margarine and jelly to top it off. I could polish off a half gallon of orange juice while consuming a couple of bagels slathered with cream cheese for a Sunday breakfast.

Even as I got older, I continued these high carbohydrate eating patterns. During my undergraduate years, I regularly consumed tacos or meatball parmesan heroes—often at 2 a.m. Yet, during that time, I was able to control my weight through a variety of intra-mural sports. During graduate school, my life became more sedentary, and I began to gain weight. While studying alone, I would consume a whole pizza; surely not a way to maintain a healthy physique. A snack could consist of two or three jelly donuts. For a solid ten-year period, I struggled to balance weight gain with jogging, gym memberships, and various diets. Fortunately, those activities kept my weight in control.

Near the end of this time period, I became engaged to a lovely woman, Ellen. My personal life gave me the greatest satisfaction I could ever imagine. In Ellen, I found a wonderful spouse who is truly a love and life partner. As we joined our lives together, she became aware of my weight issues and was always helpful by cooking healthy meals and by encouraging exercise. However, we were both busy working people who didn't like to cook, and we both enjoyed dining out at various restaurants quite often. As a consequence, we both became aware of the need to diet and exercise, which we did together.

As time progressed, I began to achieve many of my professional dreams. Central to my goals was to become a college professor, and a period of applications and interviews ensued. Fortunately, I was offered a full-time teaching position in the Ph.D. Program in Clinical & School Psychology at Hofstra University in Long Island, NY, which I gladly accepted. Once there, I dug into all of the challenges that such a position demands. Primarily, I prepared lectures for my course assignments and began to develop a program of research. Sitting, reading, studying, and writing became my devotion. University life was very sedentary, and my weight slowly rose.

Pregnancy did me in altogether. This might sound odd. I was totally overjoyed when Ellen first told me that we were going to have a baby. Wow! I was to be a father. I never really considered how my wife's pregnancy could affect me physically, but it did. As Ellen ate for two, so did I. In a well known phenomenon called "sympathetic weight gain," I added a tremendous amount of bulk to my frame and became obese. As Ellen lost her extra pounds following the birth of our son, Benjamin, I lost none of mine. Three years later, we had another pregnancy and the birth of my daughter Leah, which led to more weight struggles for me.

Being overweight was a major contributor to many health problems. My obesity began to impact my health in a serious way. I became borderline hypertensive and felt short of breath just walking up stairs. Later on, I found myself out of breath walking on flat ground and even had difficulty standing up from a chair. Playing games or sports outdoors with my children had its challenges. Daily medications became part of my life. In a move that others have characterized as "desperate," I had a stomach lap band bariatric surgery. I believe that this move saved my life. In the years following that procedure, I lost forty-five pounds and felt healthier than I had in years. Still, I was not a lightweight by any means.

Avoiding My Symptoms

In my day-to-day discussions with people about diabetes, there are those occasional stories of people who had no thought whatsoever, no warning signs or symptoms, that something was amiss with their blood sugar. That was definitely not my experience.

As the human body ages, we know that we may experience many common changes. It is not unusual for many people to begin to need reading glasses in their forties or to have occasional difficulty remembering certain names or words. Sleeping patterns may change; mine certainly did.

I used to be able to go to sleep and remain sleeping until I awoke refreshed. In January of 2005, this pattern began to change. On occasion, I found it necessary to awaken to urinate during the night. This did not seem that unusual, and I was not concerned. Over a series of weeks, the pattern became more regular, and I began to wonder if I had developed a bad behavioral pattern: that is, a bad habit of waking up. Some nights, I tried to resist getting out of bed and hoped that I would be able to sleep, but I could not. When I went to the bathroom, I always voided.

As the weeks progressed, I began to awaken twice on some nights. This seemed odd at first, but quick trips to the bathroom allowed me to return to my much needed sleep. I thought about the advice that I had always given to parents with children who wet their beds at night: restrict fluid intake for a couple of hours before bedtime, and void before going to sleep. I took my own advice. However, I still needed to get up on a few nights regardless of adhering to this plan. A few nights became many, and then eventually it became every night. Might this be a problem? I didn't think so. Denial is powerful!

Changes were occurring to my body during the day as my nighttime awakenings were increasing. Drinking plenty of fluids was a common pattern for me; it often went along with a pattern of eating a lot of food. Many diets train participants to drink many glasses of water daily as a way of filling the body and flushing out impurities. Without realizing it, I began consuming larger amounts of water from the department cooler. However, I would never have described myself as feeling particularly thirsty, a typical question asked of potential patients with diabetes.

While sitting in my office, I suddenly developed intense urges to urinate. The urges would come on rapidly and without warning. The profound sensation told me that if I didn't get to the bathroom NOW, I would have an accident at any moment. My pattern of walking to the restroom was replaced with speed walking and even running in order to relieve myself. Sometimes it felt that urine might even be trickling out of me as I moved. When I reached the bathroom, I might have had a considerable amount of urine to void, or I might have almost none. This frightened me, and soon I believed that something was wrong with my kidneys or bladder. During this period, I convinced myself that there was no need to see anybody about this problem; I thought it would just go away, heal itself. Denial is powerful!

At night, my sleep became more frequently disturbed. On many nights, I awoke three times to urinate. During the day, I would be in the midst of a meeting when I would suddenly excuse myself and run to relieve myself. In trying to take control of what was happening, I tried to collect some data by timing the duration of my urination. What was happening to me?

Having worked closely with physicians in hospitals, I knew quite a bit about human anatomy and physiology. So I played physician and tried to consider possible diagnoses. Could this be a urinary tract infection? Was I having some problem with the bladder sphincter muscle? Denial kept me going for some time.

I was unwilling to consider the big diagnosis, yet I knew it was there. Here was the formula I knew, but did not want to confront: family history of diabetes + overweight + sedentary lifestyle + drinking large amounts of fluids + strong urinary urges = DIABETES! But did I have diabetes? No. I had a urinary tract infection. Denial is very powerful!

The nighttime awakenings were now occurring every night, and I never felt fresh and replenished in the morning. The daytime urges got stronger and more frequent. I still tried to convince myself that this problem was due to a bladder infection that somehow would fix itself. My functioning at the university was beginning to suffer because I had difficulty concentrating on my teaching and students. It finally struck me that I could no longer avoid going to get help. The cumulated discomfort and fear that I felt finally overcame my avoidance of confronting the unknown. The result of this struggle was simple; I called up and made an appointment with my physician, still hoping for that diagnosis of urinary tract infection.

Waaahhhh!

If I had been logical in any way while driving back from my physician's office that day, I would have been relieved. Basically I had been told that diabetes was a manageable condition and that my sleep problems and urinary urges would go away once my blood sugar level came down. But I was not in a logical frame of mind.

Instead, I cried like a newborn baby in that car. I cried for the life that I had known and the foods that I could no longer eat. I cried for what I had done to myself; after all, I'm a smart guy and should have seen this coming. Why didn't I control myself, my eating, and my weight? I cried for the unknown future and for my death, which I presumed would arrive very soon. I let these emotions pour out as I considered my new life with diabetes. Later, I shared my thoughts and raw emotion with Ellen, who comforted me. Now the newborn had to figure out how to crawl and walk all over again.

A Healthy Re-birth

One needs to eat to sustain life. It's an obvious fact. I knew that I had to eat, but somehow differently. There was great value in seeing a Certified Diabetes Educator. This is where one can learn how to jumpstart one's life having diabetes. After learning how to use my new "best friend," the blood glucose meter, I had a short course on how to approach eating. Surprisingly, it did not involve a thousand "don'ts" or prohibitions about "evil foods," but rather stressed balance, proportion, and thoughtful experimentation.

I learned to try out foods to determine what would work best for my metabolism. The proper sizing of food portions became a skill I eventually mastered. Learning to understand food labels and to shop for healthier food products became a regular part of life. My tongue had become sensitized as a keen sugar detector. In restaurants, I assertively inquired about whether food items such as sauces or salad dressings contained sugar. I was not shy about asking for alternatives or changes to the food that I ordered.

My new eating patterns were surprising to me. Following my emotional breakdown, I had thought that my life would be reduced to rubble because I couldn't eat what I wanted. (There was that thinking again—the baby crying for satisfaction.) All food would be bland, tasteless, and unsatisfying. How wrong I was!

In general, I have become a mindful eater, a person who is keenly aware of what I eat. Every bite of food I ingest is my choice. I don't eat if I'm not hungry or if others are being "food pushers" for whatever reasons. I am responsible for having snacks that are healthy for me, but I don't make others feel guilty for what they want to eat. For example, I find joy in being with my family in an ice cream shop or while they enjoy dessert in a restaurant. I can find satisfaction in tasting a single forkful of cake without needing a portion. I am in control of my destiny.

Life Gets Better

Seven years have elapsed since my diagnosis of type 2 diabetes, and I have embraced my life as a person with diabetes. There is little doubt that I am healthier today than I was years ago. I have slowly lost an additional twenty-five pounds and continue to lose more at my own pace. I can find healthy, satisfying, and delicious food to eat wherever I may be. I am never anxious about food or eating. Those initial fears of a horrible life with diabetes simply don't exist. They are irrational fears not based in any reality.

A life with diabetes can have challenges. Using the blood glucose meter is important to me for feedback regarding my food and activity interactions. For example, I have learned that sugar levels vary tremendously in tomato sauces, and as a consequence, I now know restaurants at which I should avoid a red sauce. Illnesses affect glucose levels, as do some of the medications to treat them. I have had my diabetes medications adjusted or changed, and I now go regularly for physician visits and have diagnostic tests because I want to. I am not a "perfect" eater. At times, I eat a little too much of this or that. At other times, I skip a meal and find myself listless later on. Yet I am aware of those behaviors and keep regulation of my sugar as a priority. As a person with type 2 diabetes, dietary control is critical, since I can't add a unit of insulin to compensate for a high-carbohydrate meal.

Ellen and I will celebrate a marriage milestone soon, twenty-five years together, sharing the ups and downs of life. I couldn't imagine what this past quarter of a century would have been like without her as part of my life. Our "babies" are well on their way to finding their own careers and interests. Ben is earning his masters in Computer Science while Leah is seriously considering becoming an English professor. While their academic achievements always make their mother and me proud, we are overjoyed just through the knowledge that our children are really friendly, thoughtful, dependable, and caring young adults.

My career at Hofstra has blossomed; I rose through the academic ranks and tenure to achieve the titles of Professor and Director of the Ph.D. Program in Clinical Psychology. Following a lengthy examination process, I was awarded board certification, recognizing my clinical expertise in Cognitive and Behavioral Therapy, by the American Board of Professional Psychology. I have published my research in scholarly journals and books and have literally traveled around the world lecturing, most recently in Greece, Taiwan, Russia, Canada, and Romania. Throughout all of this, my diabetes has been a non-issue with a minor exception: I have had to learn to say "no sugar please" in a number of foreign languages.

My Sweet Leah

I cried again.

As the Spring 2012 semester began, Leah, now a nineteen-year-old freshman, began to complain about feeling ill. During a brief trip home, Ellen and I discussed her health and were determined to have Leah receive a thorough examination. At her transitional age, we decided that it was time to leave her pediatrician's care, and we made an appointment with an internist, which unfortunately would require a two-week delay. After listening closely to my daughter, I suggested giving her a quick blood glucose test that further aroused my suspicions. In a memorable phone call a few days later, Leah was extremely distraught and frustrated about the weeks of not feeling well, asserting that the university and its food were "killing" her. Two days later, we were at her pediatrician's office for an emergency morning appointment where my suspicion was confirmed. My baby was diagnosed with type 1 diabetes.

In the whirlwind that followed, we immediately went to my endocrinologist's office where Leah was examined and had her blood drawn for analysis. Afterwards, she was instructed on how to inject insulin, and I recall the stoic quiet and shock of this experience as it appeared on her colorless face; as it silently ripped me apart inside.

After hours with no rest or food, we finally returned home in the late afternoon, just in time to receive a phone call from the doctor's office. The results of her blood work were in, and Leah needed to go immediately to the emergency room. After hours of waiting and emergency tests, Leah was admitted to a critical care unit. Her blood glucose levels were found to be dangerously out of balance; she was dehydrated and was in a severe state of *diabetic ketoacidosis*.

As Ellen and I drove home that chilly March morning at 2:30 a.m., tears welled in my eyes again. The image of Leah alone in a room—tubes in her arm, her face ashen—remained in my head. I broke down and cried. What had I done to my daughter? How unfair was this to her? She was so young and now had to bear this burden. This was all due to my "bad genes."

Leah has come a long way in a short period of time, and so have I. Besides regaining her health, she has really learned how to regulate her glucose and adjust insulin; and she does so faithfully. What's particularly amazing to me is that she is able to do it all despite being a person who used to feel faint just having her blood drawn. She is doing so well that she is now a candidate for an insulin pump and will probably transition to one shortly. I can now recognize that I did not do anything to her purposely. Genetics are not controllable. Like me, she is taking control of her eating and her life.

My Sweet Life

My diabetes, my sugar problem, has served as a wake-up call for me. I want to live a healthy, long life, and diabetes has become a motivator to eat well and take care of myself. I also try to look out for those whom I love, as well. Before Leah was diagnosed, I tried to gently influence food choices for my independently-thinking children. Benjamin became well aware of sugar content in many beverages and now knows that consuming *excess amounts* of fruit juice, no matter how natural, is not a healthy choice. He is aware of fats in foods and has recently joined a gym. Leah and I now regularly discuss carbohydrates and sugars.

As we age, we learn to appreciate our lives so much more. There are many people who suffer from debilitating conditions, accidents, and fatal illnesses. I am fortunate to be alive and healthy in an age when a condition like diabetes is manageable. Yes—a manageable condition! I have taken control of my diabetes. Denial and avoidance are not necessary for me anymore. Diabetes doesn't define me—rather, it is just a part of my sweet life.

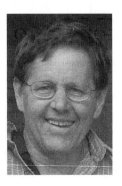

Photo credit by Brian Wright

CHAPTER 18   *by Bob Scheidt*

Living with the Dragon of Diabetes

I discovered that I had type 1 diabetes when I was eighteen years old, a few months after starting college. During the first thirty years of living with this disease, I often referred to the threat of complications and the vitality-zapping highs and lows as "battling the dragon of diabetes." As J. R. R. Tolkien wrote in *The Hobbit*, "It does not do to leave a live dragon out of your calculations, if you live near him."

So if diabetes were a dragon, surely I could not ignore it. It lived within me. I had seen too many examples of people who did not factor this disease into their calculations. In no time, the dragon could breathe fire across a scorched earth, leaving behind a loss of limbs, kidneys, and eyesight. Death could come from a bodily shutdown of systems due to either *hypoglycemia* (low blood sugar) or *hyperglycemia* (high blood sugar). I have seen friends and relatives sacrificed to the dragon. When I took to the road for the Walk Across America, it naturally followed that I thought of it as a quest to not necessarily slay the dragon but merely to control its destructive fire.

Over the last ten years or so, my thinking has evolved to where I can now frame my diabetes in more positive and poetic terms. I have come to realize that I probably accomplished many things that I might otherwise not have done had the dragon of diabetes not been stalking me. I think writer Ranier Maria Rilke summed it up best in *Letters to a Young Poet*: "Perhaps all the dragons in our lives are princesses who are only waiting to see us act, just once, with beauty and courage." I still think, at times, of living with diabetes as a quest and crusade to control this dragon, but I also understand that she, as princess, has come to teach me to act with beauty and courage.

Tough Stuff First

I've gone through some tough times in my life. I've accepted them, dealt with them, and recovered from them. From most of those tough times, I've also learned many things. With that in mind, before I begin to tell my story, I would like to list all of the major accidents, diseases, and complications that I've experienced during my thirty-nine years of living with diabetes. As in life, I will not dwell on the tough times, but will instead move on to the more positive aspects of my journey.

In my fifty-seven years of living, I have broken my right arm twice and my left arm once (basketball, climbing, and falling while hiking). I have broken my right leg twice, thirty years between breaks, the breaks being three inches apart (car accident and bicycle accident). My nose was broken four times, my ribs once, my face smashed-in after a fall into a streetlight pole during a low blood glucose seizure. When I was twenty-three years old, a huge St. Bernard mauled my face, lion-style, ripping my lower lip to where it hung loosely past my chin, causing a massive loss of blood. It took seventy stitches to recover, along with plastic surgery, and I still bear four scars to this day.

I have had insulin-dependent diabetes for nearly forty years. For the middle ten of those years, I gave five injections a day, and for the last sixteen, I have been on an insulin pump. For four years, I have had hypothyroidism, or underactive thyroid disease. Three years ago, I underwent open-heart surgery for three clogged arteries, which were successfully by-passed. The heart disease was a byproduct of both my diabetes and a family history of such maladies (my father died of a heart attack, and my mother had a crippling stroke).

To add to all of that, I have *hypoglycemia unawareness*, which has led to some nasty low blood glucose seizures. I have been tested numerous times by neurologists who were concerned that I had seizured even though my low blood sugars were not quite low enough for that kind of seizure. Part of their concern was that my father had suffered from epileptic seizures since he was a child. Several years ago, I started battling extreme seasonal allergies, which for me caused insulin resistance. I am allergic to trees, grass, and weeds, yet I spend most of my time, in both work and play, outdoors.

I realize that this sounds like a lot of bad stuff. But here is the thing: all of that tough stuff has not kept me from doing what I've wanted to do. And most of the stuff that I've wanted to do has been physical, including my business. I've rarely missed work, and I made up what I did miss by working overtime when I was healthy. I've run and walked many marathons and ultra-marathons and traveled extensively, on foot and bicycle, all over the North American continent. I have been married for thirty-six years and have put two daughters through college. It wasn't easy, but with the help of my family, a team of healthcare professionals, and the gift of a positive attitude, I have gotten to this point in time still fairly healthy. And soon, I will embark on a 2,650-mile pilgrimage, on foot, across Europe.

The Beginnings of Mostly Good Stuff

I was born in February, 1955 in Allentown, PA. I lived for most of my young life in a semi-rural part of southeastern Pennsylvania. The most important factor in my childhood was location. Our house was surrounded on three sides by eastern deciduous forests. To the west were a few acres of trees, whose significance lay in the fact that they offered a young boy a place in which to play, sleep, and learn fairly close to home. Eventually, I graduated to the fields and woodlands that stretched for miles to the south. The fields were divided by stone walls built hundreds of years ago.

After a mile or so, the land started to rise, an ascent of only a couple of hundred feet, but enough to provide a 270-degree view to the north. There lay a wall of blue mountains, about twenty-five miles as the crow flies, part of the Kittatinny Ridge. I looked with amazement at those mountains—they were only about 1,700 feet high, but to a young boy feeling the first pangs of a hunger for adventure, they could well have been the Karakorum Range of Pakistan. And then came the knowledge that, along that ridge, ran a 2,000 mile trail—a trail that, if you went south. would bring you to Georgia and. if you went north, would take you to Maine. I was looking out at what was close to the midpoint of the Appalachian Trail.

Behind our house, to the northeast, was my favorite place in my then-limited world. A hike of one mile brought me to a swift-flowing little stream that continued flowing through a deep, dark pine wood. Above the creek and pines towered a small peak covered in immense boulders. From the top I could see the village of Bowers, and farther on the borough of Kutztown. It was exciting to hike up there on cold, clear nights and watch the sunset fade while the lights of the valley slowly switched on. One January night, during a whiteout blizzard, I crawled one mile over eight-foot drifts to the pine forest, carrying a full backpack. Using an ancient stone wall as a wind block, I stamped out a tent platform and slept out in -20° F wind chills. During summers, the creek was useful for catching snakes, lizards, and frogs. I had quite a collection, but returned most of them to the creek when my mom was repeatedly frightened by reptiles and amphibians in her wash basket. I was a great outdoorsman but a lousy carpenter, and the cages I built leaked specimens all over our basement.

All through those years, I was growing strong and fearless and spending many days and nights in the woods. However, sometimes I did play a variety of sports with my younger brothers on a field next to our house. My brothers' athletic abilities eventually eclipsed mine, especially as I spent more and more time traipsing through the fields and forests. My flagging energy during our basketball games was perhaps my first sign of diabetes. I just couldn't keep up with my brothers, even though they were three and four years younger than I. And while all of us were tall and thin, I started losing more weight and experiencing blurry vision.

At the time, my girlfriend's mother was the first to guess diabetes, which was then confirmed by our family doctor. In fact, that was as far as you got in 1973. The family doctor did the blood test (630 mg/dL blood glucose), taught me how to give insulin (one shot of NPH a day in the morning), and had me come to his office every Saturday at 6 a.m. to draw blood for a glucose test. I remember how disheartened I was on those mornings when all of the other people getting their blood tested were much older than I. The doctor had already told me that I would live only twenty to thirty more years, and that most of those days would involve a tragic loss of limbs, eyesight, and kidney function. I was eighteen years old and now had a demoralizing vision of a life diminished. The doctor also told me that I should take it easy and try to avoid any infection-causing injuries.

Now here is where I discovered that I had a very strong will and an optimistic view of life. I just downgraded the optimism a tad and kept right on doing what I had been doing. I spent my days working in the mornings at a car wash, going to community college in the afternoons and nights, and dreaming of the weekends when my girlfriend and I would head to the mountains to hike, bike, backpack, and climb. I had to make a few adjustments in my lifestyle, but I could still go on adventures. I now realized that the woods of my boyhood had served their purpose, helping to make me strong and teaching me countless lessons.

The time had come for growing up and moving on. Beyond my own little world was a much bigger world waiting to be explored. Right now, that was all that mattered.

Walking Through a Minefield of Health

In 1974, my girlfriend, Nancy (still the same girlfriend, and eventually wife, at any point in this story), and I were accepted to Penn State University. I would be a sophomore, and Nancy a freshman. After lousy-to-middling grades in high school, I had proven myself in community college and was eager to begin studying in the journalism program at Penn State.

The summer before classes started, Nancy and I decided to take the long drive across Pennsylvania to look for an apartment and part-time jobs for the fall semester. On the drive back home, however, our future was forever altered when we were involved in a horrible five-car pileup that amazingly left no one dead, but caused crippling injuries for Nancy and me. I couldn't walk or work for a year and had to put off college because of finances. I tried to keep fit by doing upper body exercises and working my way up to several miles on crutches until I had armpit blisters. Thus began a string of health problems, some of which were listed earlier. I was in the hospital repeatedly.

Once again, the constant pitfalls of that time did not cause me to downgrade my optimism. I think I was still in a *honeymoon phase* with my diabetes, and there were no blood glucose meters for testing anyway. It was hard to tell if my blood sugar was high or low. All I knew was that I still had huge energy reserves. When I finally recovered from the accident, I started apprenticing for a house painter/decorator and made up for lost time by climbing and backpacking as much as I could. In 1976, Nancy and I got married. In 1977, I was away for forty-two weekends of the year (half with Nancy), all over the northeastern U.S. and New England. We honeymooned on the Appalachian Trail in Shenandoah National Park, then took a three-week trip to Utah and Colorado, where we climbed three 14,000-foot peaks and backpacked throughout Rocky Mountain National Park.

In the ensuing years, we fell in love with the Adirondack Mountains of New York, the White Mountains of New Hampshire, the Green Mountains of Vermont, and especially the Allegheny Mountains of north-central Pennsylvania. I cherish the memory of how I managed my diabetes on the trails, taking extra supplies of everything and putting my insulin bottles in cold springs after we reached camp.

From all of the heavy climbing and descending with a fully loaded pack while wearing bulky five-pound boots, I developed massive tree-trunk calves and thighs. My upper body was wraith-like, my body fat extremely low. Most weekends, we arrived home from the mountains late Sunday night, removed the dirty clothes and pots and pans from our backpacks, and left everything else packed up so that the next Friday, we only had to add clean clothes, dishes, and food. It was one of the most exciting times of my life. All the hard physical work of my job and the medical problems that popped up were soon forgotten when the maps were spread out on the apartment floor as we planned where to climb next. We felt that we were following in the footsteps of a long list of explorers throughout history, training for the future when we too would be remembered by the next generation.

The Symbolism of Maps

Upon opening my lunch box, looking in my car, or walking into my house, one would notice two constants: diabetes supplies and maps. The latter were the driving force behind helping me concentrate on controlling my disease. If I continued to discipline myself and kept up on the educational dimensions of diabetes, I could keep on living an active life. That was difficult because the 1970s were still the "dark ages" of diabetes control.

The maps caused my pulse to race as I followed the contours and elevations, traced the blue squiggle of rivers, and sought out destinations old and new. What really quickened my pulse was finding an unexplored spot on the map and making plans to explore it. These plans included making equipment lists, doing reconnaissance, figuring out mileages, and putting together a team of dreamers just like myself. The maps were the catalyst.

Years later, my wife sometimes resented maps because they took me away from home. We joked about how, during nights of restlessness, I would sometimes go downstairs and sit at the kitchen table poring over a map. She would awaken to find the bed empty and start down the steps. I would hear her coming down and quickly grab an old *Playboy* magazine that I kept for just this purpose, shoving the map into the folds of the magazine. When my wife would round the corner, she would be foiled by the map-less kitchen table. According to my friend Dave, "Maps are the new porn."

My Life List

The 1980s brought innovations in diabetes control for me in the form of three major factors. The first was the advent of endocrinologists, doctors trained in diabetes care. Mine was Dr. Larry Merkle, and he had had good results with a few other athletes and adventurers. He introduced me to number two on the list, which was multiple shots of short-acting insulin combined with two shots of long-acting NPH. This freed me up from the time constraints of having to live by the dictates of NPH's peaks and valleys. It helped me put on muscle, something I was struggling to do, especially on my upper body. Number three on the list was a godsend of technology: self-testing blood glucose meters. No more Saturday morning visits to my doctor's office. With those innovations came a sense of a possibly longer life span. I started to realize that people with diabetes could defy the odds.

Back when I was fourteen, I remember going with my parents to visit a friend of theirs. It was a Sunday afternoon, and I would rather have been in my beloved woods. I wandered off to an office/library down the hall and perused the books and magazines. And right there it was, waiting for me to stumble upon it: a magazine article on John Goddard, an adventurer who had made a life list (an early precursor of the bucket list). On it he had listed: climb Mount Everest, raft the Nile, run a sub-five-minute mile, read the entire Encyclopedia Britannica, etc. His list eventually went past one hundred items.

I was entranced, and immediately started making my own list. Since that time, I have crossed off several listings and added some new ones. I still have my original list, though it is worn, faded, and practically unreadable. Still, I take it with me when I give presentations, especially at camps for kids with diabetes. I hope they can sense its iconic worth to me just in seeing it and touching it. It became a beacon for me during hard times, for once again I knew that I had to be healthy to continue the life on that list. In the 1980s, especially, some of those items on my list spurred me on to some of the most difficult, yet meaningful, accomplishments of my life.

The Long, Slow, Ultra-Distance Shuffle

In the late 1970s, I started running to keep in shape for climbing and backpacking. It started with a 10K run sponsored by the Saucony Shoe Company located in Kutztown, PA, across the street from where my wife and I had just moved into our first house. Nothing really exciting happened at the race. I had fun, made some new friends, felt that little bit of runner's high. I definitely enjoyed backpacking a lot more, yet somehow I was sucked into the great running boom. It swept me along race after race, going so far as to sweep me to out-of-state races, eventually overnight trips to major races with long histories. It seriously cut into my hiking, since the distances got progressively longer. In only one year, I was running marathons, then using marathons to train for ultra-marathons, then running all-day ultra-marathons to train for multi-day ultra-marathons. Now don't get me wrong, I wasn't a fast or talented runner. I was actually more like a plodder, with a developing wrestler's upper body and muscular legs. I did, however, have great endurance. I could literally run all day and night. My best marathon time was 3:30, and my best fifty-mile race was done in eight hours.

Along with all of the training I had to do, other priorities were developing. We had our first daughter, Adrienne, in 1983 and our second, Amberly, in 1988. In 1986, I started my own house-painting company, Bob Scheidt's Ultra Painting, specializing in the exterior and interior of churches, some with difficult-to-reach steeples. My mountain climbing knowledge and equipment certainly came in handy. One of the ways that I got in some extra-distance mileage was to take my infant daughters out for long midnight walks, especially when they were colicky. They always settled down once I got moving, creating a bond between father and daughter and helping me win some arguments with my wife about theories of nomads in constant movement. I also started a 5 a.m. paper route that required me to walk five miles each day carrying two huge sacks of papers. It was great resistance training, and I got paid for doing a workout. I continued that for five years. Thank God that I was relatively healthy during the 1980s!

I did occasionally get some minor over-use symptoms from all of the mileage. My 6-foot-1-inch, 190-pound frame created a lot of force on every footfall. Since the distances kept escalating, I started to mix in some walking. Most ultra-distance athletes did. I eventually completed twenty marathons and thirty ultra-marathons. Using bicycling as cross-training, I also completed a 24-hour bike race.

In the upper reaches of the sport of the ultra-distances was the six-day race. So, after running/walking several 24-hour races and one 48-hour race, I decided to try my hand at a six-day event. Obviously, most of my family, friends, and doctors thought that it was insanity. However, my endocrinologist, Dr. Merkle, thought that it would be challenging but achievable.

I would now proclaim myself to be a pure walker, no running, and I would have access to carbohydrates, insulin, and my blood glucose meter every quarter mile. Another advantage was that my youngest brother Craig would be by my side every step of the way (yes, he does take after his older brother when it comes to doing crazy stuff like this). I would also have friends and family there to act as my handlers, and all were schooled in the dangers of diabetes. So it was a calculated craziness.

One of the problems with the race was the heat and humidity of a New Jersey summer mixed with the shade-less black cinders of a quarter-mile track, in which I, and twenty-five others, would circle, hamster-like, round and round for six straight days and nights. Oh, we slept—problem is, it was a total of two to three broken hours a night, some of it while sleepwalking around the track. It was late June of 1987 when my brother and I completed the Edward Payson Weston Six-Day Race with a total of 274 miles, finishing tied for twelfth place. I don't actually know if any other person with diabetes had walked that far in six days at that point in history (a few have gone beyond since), but it felt as if I was the first. I had no problems with my diabetes, though a few nasty blisters were cautiously watched and kept at bay by a team of podiatry students in a trailer beside the track. This experience surely prepared them well for the practice of seeing patients with diabetes who had foot problems, even if most would not be self-inflicted!

The Roads of the North American Continent Beckon

In the 1990s I looked for a new high. A strange hybrid of my previous avocations started to take form in my consciousness. I still felt the pull of wilderness trails, yet craved my new love of walking long distances. So I merged the two and became a long-distance trekker, which I played by my own rules and created my own events. I had never felt comfortable in the role of competitor. I lacked finesse and aggressiveness. Soon, I even came up with a new description of what I was searching for. I found the word *aesthete*, which in Greek means "someone who searches for beauty."

I was no longer just an athlete, but also an aesthete. Just as I had always done when I backpacked, I would continue to search for beauty. The beauty of the landscapes, the beauty of a body in motion, the beauty of wildlife, and now something new—the beauty of the people I would meet along the way. I would pick out a piece of the United States, map out a route, and cover thirty to thirty-five miles a day on foot. I would carry a light pack with medical supplies, a change of clothes, foul-weather gear, and a bunch of snacks. I would stay in hostels, barns, fire company quarters, motels, and friends' homes—whoever could put me up for the night while I passed through their area. I would perform both planned and impromptu talks on the connection between exercise and diabetes health. I would come into communities and host bake sales, walk-a-thons, raffles, and T-shirt sales to raise money for several diabetes charities. I even did a few of those fundraisers for other diseases, such as cancer and multiple sclerosis.

I walked across Pennsylvania, both east to west and north to south. I walked up Virginia and Maryland. And I walked from San Francisco to Los Angeles along the west coast. It was a time of high adventure, and I reveled in the raw exuberance of this reinvented form of travel. The time had now come to walk across the country as a whole: one route, west to east, across the raw bulge and bulk of the American continent.

In 1996, after twenty-three years of diabetes, my control seemed to hit a plateau. I was doing what I had always done, using a holistic idea of diabetes care. Physical, mental, spiritual. Mind, body, spirit. I viewed it as a square, the four points being medication (for me, insulin), diet, exercise, and spirituality. All of that was still a consistent factor in my diabetes control, and all of those points were getting better and better with education and technology. My plateau was thus quite perplexing. So I looked to a higher degree of technology to help me out: I started on an insulin pump. The results were immediate, probably because some of my problems stemmed from timing issues. For instance, the effects of the *dawn phenomenon* were immediately softened by a slowly building surge of pre-morning insulin. (The *dawn phenomenon* is the term used to describe an abnormal early-morning increase in blood glucose—usually between 2 a.m. and 8 a.m.) However, over the years, the real value of the pump came from the lifestyle advantage that it gave people with crazy schedules such as me. My pump let me tailor my insulin flow to better fit that sometimes hectic schedule.

The Walk Across America for Diabetes came directly from that original life list that I had made as a boy of fourteen years old. It was something that I had always dreamed about, both daydreams and nighttime dreams. As I walked the paths of my boyhood forests, I often pictured a slice of faraway American landscapes, imagining those landscapes, almost conjuring them into being. My nighttime dreams were of the Great Plains. One cannot walk across America without hitting the Great Plains somewhere. Interest in Native American cultures became prominent in those dreams of big skies, rolling thunderheads, and undulating hills. And when I finally crossed those American landscapes, I was amazed at how close those dreams were to the reality. All was foreshadowed.

In 1997, I drove my just-purchased 1977 eighteen-foot logo-plastered motorhome across the continent, from eastern Pennsylvania to just north of Seattle, Washington. I stepped out the back door of that motorhome on a warm, early June morning at Bay Shore State Park. I dipped my walking pole into the salty water, turned around, and looked east to what would consume me for most of the next three years.

My plan was to walk for two months each year, 1,150 miles, one-third of the continent in each bite. This plan would allow me to work ten months of the year to keep the bills paid back home and also give me time to plan the next section of the walk. I tried to schedule a presentation every day, though in some of the more remote areas of the route, that would prove difficult. The American Association of Diabetes Educators (AADE) and the Lions Club International helped a lot. Some days, I did a presentation at a senior center at noon, a school at 3 p.m., and a Lions Club at 7 p.m. I still had to walk twenty-five miles each day and keep up tight blood glucose control. It was grueling. But I was in the groove of a lifetime, knowing full well that this was what I was born to do.

I was in the early stages of understanding that my walking was much more than exercise, diabetes control, or adventure. I now saw that walking was my art form. Over time and miles, I've further developed this theory, but to keep it simple, I use as an example an encounter I had with a newspaper reporter. When I blurted out that walking was my art form, he seemed a bit confused. So I quickly thought up two analogies that I still treasure to this day: "I want to walk like John Coltrane played the saxophone. I want to walk like Miles Davis played the trumpet."

Over the next three years, there were many highlights as I walked the roads and trails of the continent: the heavy snows and jagged peaks of the North Cascades in Washington; the new friends I met on Native American reservations who inspired me deeply; the contrast between the Rocky Mountains and the Great Plains of Montana. In 1998, I drove back to where I had ended the previous year in the Badlands of North Dakota and headed east on foot once more. Eventually, I came to my first Great Lake. I arrived on the hills above Duluth and saw, shimmering in the late afternoon sun, Lake Superior. I was so enchanted that I went off route and walked up its western shore for days. Lake Michigan, Lake Huron, and Lake Erie followed, all vast inland oceans with waves and shorebird life.

Then, leaving Cleveland, I ran out of Great Lakes and continued into my home state of Pennsylvania. Now that I was back east, I noticed one of my least favorite of atmospheric conditions: humidity. In Pennsylvania, the rivers were my companions, most notably the Susquehanna, the Lehigh, and the Delaware. I reached the Atlantic Ocean on Memorial Day 1999, where a busload of friends and family, accompanied by Miss America, Nicole Johnson, walked the last two miles with me. After a speech, Nicole crowned me warrior king in the fight against diabetes. After reaching the ocean, I thrust my walking staff into the waves and then joined hands with twenty of my nuttier friends who ran with me into the cold Atlantic. Over the next three days, I was accompanied by

Miss New York, Deanna Herrera, on a media blitz throughout New York City, including an appearance on *The Today Show* and an interview with Ann Curry. Thus ended my grand adventure. Or did it?

A Circumambulation of the United States

During the latter stages of The Walk Across America, I posited a question to my crew: How about we continue the entire endeavor to include all three coasts and the southern border of the United States? It seemed like a natural progression. We had crossed America at the very northern of its borders. There was a real sense of closure to be able to close the loop around the circumference of the country. Most importantly, we could continue to visit hospitals, camps, villages, and reservations with our message of hope for those living with diabetes as we made our way across these new landscapes. We called it Adventure on the Rim of America. It was an audacious idea that would take another five years, more sponsorship, and more planning. Could we really pull this one off? Well, we were surely going to try!

We had two new tools in our arsenal. We had created a puppet show for kids based on the people and animals that we met along the earlier stretch of our journey. And I had further developed a set of mythical archetypes that I used as inspiration to motivate me to continue my walk during energy ebbs and bad weather. I arranged my slide show around these archetypes with the hope that they could motivate people with diabetes. The show, titled *Seven Mythical Archetypes for Diabetics to Live By*, included 1) The quest, 2) The pilgrimage, 3) Women who run with the wolves, 4) The explorer/discoverer, 5) The jester/coyote trickster/holy fool, 6) The warrior, 7) The archetype of service.

I drove back to Seattle in July of 2000, my oldest daughter, Adrienne, now able to help with the driving. This time I headed south on foot, using ferries to hop the waters between the San Juan Islands. Over the next five years, the memories piled up once more: the wild Washington coast was primal; the beauty of the Oregon coast blew me away and became my favorite place in the world—so far; we climbed the third highest peak in Oregon, South Sister; and we strolled through the deep, dark redwood forests of northern California. On Thanksgiving Day 2001, my wife, Nancy, my daughters, Amberly and Adrienne, and a few others met me on the Golden Gate Bridge. There were more wonders to behold heading south along that mightiest of oceans. Big Sur was a vortex of energy and mysticism; Los Angeles was culture shock all the way to San Diego.

Then came the deserts of the southwest. I was nervous. I had been along some form of water for more than 5,000 miles. Now there would be very few waterways to walk along until the Rio Grande. But I found the deserts extremely interesting, a stark yet constantly changing landscape of mountains and cactus. Most importantly, it had low humidity and no allergens.

In El Paso, TX, I switched to bicycle and rode to the Atlantic coast of Florida at Saint Augustine. Some highlights were Big Bend National Park, a few days of biking into northern Mexico, and the beaches of the Gulf Coast. We were now leaving the west behind, including Native American reservations. We had visited thirty-two reservations and found that, on most of them, diabetes was rampant. I biked into New Orleans in December of 2003 (pre-Hurricane Katrina), following the Mississippi River along the soon-to-be-destroyed levees. I flew to Chicago to accept the "Athlete of the Year" award at the annual DESA (Diabetes Exercise and Sports Association) conference then flew back and continued east along the Gulf in Alabama and the Florida panhandle.

The final year should have been 2004, a 1,200-mile bike/walk along the Atlantic Ocean from Atlantic City to Key West. At exactly the halfway point in Wilmington, NC, I was forced off the road by a pickup truck, and my bike and I went down on a set of railroad tracks, causing me to break my leg. I returned the next year after healing and gingerly got back on my bike, ending in Key West in December of 2005.

Crusades and Pilgrimages Await

Energy has always been at the forefront of my diabetes control. How can one maintain a constant supply of bodily energy, enough to be able to complete the many tasks at hand? Blood glucose highs and lows zap energy, and the worst of all is the rapid rise and fall from high to low and low to high. This is the day-to-day concern of people with long-term diabetes: activating enough energy to drive the crusade forward. There is also the spiritual form of energy, the one that Jesuit priest/paleontologist Pierre Teilhard de Chardin wrote of in his 1930s dispatches from the Gobi Desert, where he found the bones of Peking Man. For de Chardin, love was the greatest form of spiritual and physical energy: "Love is the most universal, the most tremendous and the most mysterious of the cosmic forces...the conclusion is always the same: love is most powerful and still the most unknown energy of the world."

My new adventure will begin on April Fool's Day of 2013. I will then begin a four-year, 2,650- mile pilgrimage on foot across the continent of Europe. Much like my previous walks, I will do a portion each year, likely 550 to 750 miles at a stretch. For most of the time, I will be following the "Way of St. James" from Budapest, Hungary, to the Atlantic Ocean in northeastern Spain. Eventually, I will continue on to Bucharest, Romania, and then to the Black Sea in Constanta, Romania. I will carry everything with me in a pack, and there will be no motorhome to count on anymore. I will be following in the footsteps of St Francis of Assisi, Charlemagne, and writer Paul Coelho. I will be crossing my second continent. That leaves only five more.

This is my destiny. This is what I was born to do. I must continue no matter what obstacles, including diabetes, lie in my path. The following quote, by Harold Thurman Whitman, carries a great deal of weight and resonance for me: "Don't ask yourself what the world needs—ask yourself what makes you come alive, and then go do it. Because what the world needs is people who have come alive."

I have learned that the dragon of diabetes does offer some inspirations for me, propelling me forward. So the goal, then, is to control the dragon, not to slay it. For it can be a positive life force. In the novel *A Game of Thrones*, author George R. R. Martin writes about the queen of a nomadic tribe, Danerys Targaryen, who wanders the fictional wastelands and contends with rebellion, drought, and starvation in a hostile land far from home. She does, however, have three dragon eggs. One night, at the low point of her life, she contemplates suicide. But the next morning she rises from the ashes, and on her shoulder is a newly born dragon, breathing fire and emitting an unearthly scream. It then becomes her life-altering challenge to harness the power of that dragon—and maybe use that power to make the world a better place.

Sound familiar? To teach you to live your life with beauty and courage: That is the power of the dragon.

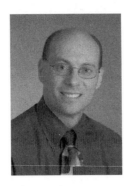

CHAPTER 19 *by Gary Scheiner, MS, CDE*

Attitude Will
Get You Everywhere

Let's get this out of the way right now. Diabetes is a pain in the butt.

I don't mean it in the literal sense. Syringes and pump infusion sets are little more than a flick on the skin. But when it comes to day-to-day living, diabetes is a general nuisance. Think about it. We have all the "usual" responsibilities—work, school, family, home, etc., and have all the tasks associated with this twenty-four-hour chronic health condition piled on top of it. But if there's one thing I've learned, it's this: *developing the right attitude is the secret to success.*

It was a hot, muggy Wednesday afternoon in Sugar Land, TX, a suburb in southwest Houston. (No, I'm not making this up.) I was at home on summer break after my freshman year of college, spending half my time drinking juice and the other half urinating it out. My energy was gone, and there was no way the Houston summer could have caused me to lose so much weight. (I had gone from 155 pounds to 117 pounds.) I was down to the last belt loop on my pants, yet they were still falling halfway down my butt. Then I saw an episode of the TV show M*A*S*H in which a character had diabetes. And guess what—he had the same symptoms! So I decided it was time to get checked out.

It was only a ten-minute drive from my family's house to the doctor's office, during which I had to make one stop to use a gas station restroom. When I got to the doctor's office, I wiped the humidity off my glasses, hit the bathroom yet again, and sat in the waiting room wishing they had a water fountain.

After a quick physical exam, blood test, and urinalysis, the doctor came back in and said nonchalantly, "Gary, I've got good news and I've got bad news. The bad news is that you have diabetes."

I have no idea what the good news was because I stopped listening at that point.

"Diabetes? What the heck was that? It can't be good if it starts with 'die'."

I remember him telling me that my blood sugar was 600-something mg/dL and that I would have to take shots of insulin and be very careful of what I ate. The thought of giving myself shots was one thing. But limiting what I ate? Was he crazy? I was an active eighteen-year-old with an over-active metabolism. The thought of limiting what I ate made me more depressed than anything else.

So off I went the same day to an endocrinologist in downtown Houston. Keep in mind that the year was 1985, so there was no HMO red tape to deal with.

"You are lucky to be diagnosed now," he told me. "We have come a long way in the treatment of diabetes. The way research is going, I'll bet that in five or ten years, there will be a cure."

I should have taken that bet.

I then met with a nurse who taught me what insulin was and why it was important to maintain my blood sugar levels. I also learned how food and exercise affected my blood sugar levels. Finally, I was instructed on how to inject insulin. I did not practice first on oranges, pillows, or teddy bears. I gave myself my very first injection, right in the stomach. It hurt—probably because I had no fat left on my body, and the syringe needles were much thicker and longer than they are today. But what hurt more was the thought of having to stick myself with needles for the rest of my life.

I was also given a bottle of test strips and taught about blood sugar testing. No meter. Just test strips. These strips had a big square box (still can't figure out how to get a square drop of blood to come out of my finger) that had to be covered with blood, blotted, and then timed before matching the color on the strip to the color chart on the bottle. Subtle differences in the blue/green color spectrum meant big differences in blood sugar, so you had to be a graphic artist to get the number right. To get a blood sample, we used a medieval torture device called an Autolet® lancet device. A disposable 25-gauge lancet was placed in the firing mechanism, which swung around at a high speed like a pendulum, stabbed your finger and made it bleed. Oh, what fun!

My first meal plan was the highlight of the whole experience. I can still remember my "generous" 2,500-calorie Exchange System diet—chock-full of fruits exchanges, vegetables exchanges, meat exchanges, milk exchanges, fat exchanges, and starch exchanges. Oh, how I hated that diet. I was hungry constantly. My first Exchange System diet meal consisted of a sandwich, a piece of fruit, a cup of milk, and a handful of chips. And there were no seconds, thirds, or fourths, as I was used to having. Today, the "diet" is totally different and is based on counting carbohydrates and matching insulin to the food, not the other way around.

A few weeks after my diagnosis, I purchased my first blood glucose meter—a Glucometer, to be exact. It weighed about a pound and was the size of a brick. The testing procedure is still etched in my brain: pendulum, then squeeze out a big "hanging" drop of blood, dab the big box on the strip, start the counter, wait one minute, blot the strip, and insert it into the meter, press the button again, and wait ninety seconds for a number to appear. And believe me, there weren't a lot of results in the 100s mg/dL.

My early insulin program presented another set of challenges: NPH and Regular insulin, at breakfast and dinner. The Regular would peak in about two hours and last about six hours; the NPH would peak in five hours and last about twelve hours. Basically, that meant that I would have to eat certain things at certain times of day; exercise (with caution) at certain times of day; sleep only at certain times because of the need to take shots at specific times; and test my blood sugar at certain times. In those days, two shots a day was the norm. So was making your life conform to your insulin regimen. Nevertheless, I was determined to not let diabetes keep me from doing anything that I set my mind to, even if it meant getting "creative" with my meal and insulin program.

Things did improve over time. I was given a "sliding scale" for my insulin so that I could do something about the highs, and my evening NPH was moved to bedtime. With all the exercise that I did, I probably had as many low blood sugars as high blood sugars, so my *glycosylated hemoglobin* (A1c) levels showed a decent overall average. But the low blood sugar reactions were becoming more frequent and more severe, especially during the night.

When I returned to college for my sophomore year (Washington University in St. Louis—home of the world's best frozen custard), I learned what it meant to get by with a little help from my friends. Before dinner, my roommates would gather to wager on my blood sugar. Everyone threw a dollar on the table; closest guess took the money. Some of them were fast learners. They would ask about the day's food and exercise before making their guesses.

Exercise and sports played a big role in helping me keep a positive attitude. I had always been into fitness, but after being diagnosed with diabetes, my passion for staying in shape reached a whole new level. Every day, I found a way to work out. If there wasn't anybody to play basketball with, I would ride my bike, jump rope, or go to the athletic complex to lift weights with members of the football and rugby teams. Unfortunately, the emotional "high" that I got from working out was often followed by blood sugar lows. To make matters worse, I was starting to lose the early warning signs of *hypoglycemia* (aka *hypoglycemia unawareness*).

Thank God for my wife, Debbie. I met her during my junior year in college and knew I would marry her after our first Valentine's Day together.

She learned a few things about diabetes and went out of her way to prepare a huge heart-shaped box filled with popcorn and pistachios. (The way to a man's heart is truly through his pancreas!)

After graduating from Washington University, we moved to Chicago. It was there that I had some of the worst low blood sugars of my life. Most came in the middle of the night. Debbie had to give me a *glucagon* injection once and had to call paramedics a few times. Those experiences really shook me up. I met with an exercise physiologist who worked at a diabetes clinic. He had diabetes himself and gave me some suggestions about eating extra food at bedtime and self-adjusting my long-acting insulin to prevent the nighttime lows after exercise. Little did he know that his impact on me went far beyond merely helping to manage my blood sugar.

You see, I went to college with every intention of becoming a doctor. Somewhere along the way, I lost interest in going to medical school. I think it had something to do with the way pre-med and medical students worked and studied themselves into oblivion. I felt that many people graduated from medical school devoid of compassion and personality. I decided that it wasn't worth that kind of sacrifice. What I hadn't decided was what I would do instead. I bounced back and forth between majors in college, and tried working in a variety of different fields after graduation—including jobs in advertising and public relations. I had the opportunity to be creative and did a great deal of writing (which I enjoyed), but it still felt like punching a clock. I just couldn't find something I was really passionate about. Something that made me excited about getting up and going to work in the morning: work that didn't feel like *work*.

That exercise physiologist opened my eyes to more than just how to balance food, exercise, and insulin. He inspired me to find a career in the diabetes field, helping others to take better care of themselves. I went to graduate school to earn a Masters degree in exercise physiology and was fortunate to land a position with the Joslin Diabetes Center's affiliate in Philadelphia. It was a place that stressed a positive, "can do" approach with all of its patients. My office was filled with fitness equipment and offered a great view of the sports complex in South Philly. Even better, the clinical team of doctors, nurses, dietitians, and psychologists taught me a great deal about flexible insulin management and every conceivable aspect of diabetes care.

Our diabetes center was fast becoming the talk of the town, but we had not yet started an insulin pump program. In 1994, I volunteered to give insulin pumping a try – mostly to give our clinicians a chance to learn how the devices worked. My first pump was a bit clunky, and the infusion set was a bent needle that I could not disconnect. But having the ability to adjust *basal* insulin levels and deliver very precise mealtime doses really helped to stabilize my blood sugar levels. For the first time in almost ten years, I could sleep past 8 a.m.

without having my blood sugar skyrocket. I could delay my lunch without my blood sugar bottoming out. And best of all, I could exercise to my heart's content without having a low blood sugar reaction in the middle of the night. In fact, I haven't had a single severe *hypoglycemic reaction* since I started using an insulin pump nearly twenty years ago.

With pump therapy came a whole new approach to dietary management: carbohydrate counting. By counting the grams of carbohydrate in my meals and snacks, I can now eat what I choose as long as I match it with the correct dose of rapid-acting insulin. Speaking of which, the introduction of rapid-acting insulin in the late 1990s worked wonders for improving after-meal blood sugar control and preventing big drops before meals. A few years ago, I began dabbling with other injectable medications designed to help control appetite and improve after-meal control: *Amylin* and GLP-1 hormones.

And then there's the latest technological innovation—continuous glucose monitors (CGMs). I began using a CGM back in 2004, when the data was "blinded" to the user and the receiver was connected to your body by way of a thick gray cable. Today's systems are sleek, wireless, and much easier to use. While far from perfect, the fact that they alert me when blood sugars are starting to creep out of range has helped me prevent many extreme highs and lows. I also love the way they provide *context* to blood sugar values. Knowing if my blood sugar is rising or falling lets me make more effective decisions.

Technology has certainly come a long way since my diagnosis. Modern high-tech pumps, sensors, meters, software, and apps may not make having diabetes worthwhile, but they have made living with it a whole lot easier. Not that walking around like a "pseudo-cyborg" is fun, but it's easy to take if you keep a sense of humor about it. Nothin' like playing "find the infusion set" with my wife!

Besides the cool gadgets, there are some good things about having diabetes. It certainly set me on a very satisfying career path, and I know it has done the same for many others who have entered the fields of medicine, nursing, dietetics, mental health, biomedical engineering, pharmaceutical sales, and nonprofit management. Today I own and direct a successful diabetes education practice called Integrated Diabetes Services. (For further information about my practice, please see the website at the conclusion of this chapter.) My team of CDEs (Certified Diabetes Educators) works with clients throughout the world via all forms of electronic communications, focusing on intensive insulin therapy and advanced self-management training. Those writing skills that I honed early in my professional career are being put to really good use. I've written five books and more than one hundred articles on all different aspects of diabetes self-management. Being on the diabetes lecture circuit has allowed me to travel to many interesting places, meet amazing people, and make some really good friends. Here are a few other potential benefits of having diabetes:

If you have to undergo a medical procedure, be thankful you have diabetes. Most medical/surgical centers give preferential treatment to people who take insulin, and schedule their procedures first.

It's easy to strike up a conversation and make new friends. Watch for people checking their blood sugar or wearing an insulin pump, or just follow the trail of glucose tablet wrappers or used test strips to find someone with whom you have a lot in common.

Market research companies *love* people with diabetes. Pharmaceutical companies and device manufacturers are constantly testing new products and marketing strategies, and they need actual users of the products for focus groups, surveys, and sampling. And the pay is pretty good!

Now I would *never* do this myself, but many people use their diabetes as a sort of "get out of jail free card." If you did something wrong, it's easy to claim "my blood sugar was low" or something to that effect. And if you just don't feel like doing chores or sitting in a boring meeting, you can always excuse yourself because you have to take a shot, check your blood sugar, or eat.

Some businesses even provide preferential treatment to people with diabetes. The last thing a restaurant owner wants is for someone to have a *hypoglycemic* seizure in the lobby. If there's a wait for a table, whip out your syringes and let the manager know that you're at risk for a severe low blood sugar reaction if you're not seated soon. You'll be surprised how quickly they find a table for you. Likewise, amusement park owners don't want to risk a wrongful death lawsuit, so most are happy to provide special passes to people with diabetes (and their party) that allows them to bypass the long, hot waiting lines.

Most businesses and organizations are compelled by the Americans with Disabilities Act to provide special accommodations to people with diabetes. Not that I have ever considered diabetes to be a "disability," but if it helps get us a few breaks at work or school, why not? We put up with a lot living with diabetes.

So, yes, diabetes is a pain in the butt. But it's *our* pain in the butt. So as long as we're stuck with it, we might as well take care of it... and have some fun along the way. If there's one thing that I've learned after all these years, it's that everyone has to face challenges. Being equipped with all the tools and expert guidance in the world doesn't cut it. It's your attitude—keeping a sense of humor, looking for answers, and not letting anything get in your way—that really makes the difference.

www.integrateddiabetes.com

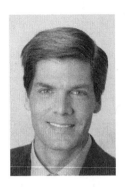

CHAPTER 20   *by Benno C. Schmidt III*

What's Wrong with Me? Diagnosis and Triumph

This is the story about how I got diabetes while in college and how that diagnosis and living with diabetes doesn't *define* me, but certainly is part of nearly *all* my decisions, mundane or momentous. Perhaps most importantly, it is about how I turned diabetes into something positive and how I learned about my body. I've been fortunate to have met, befriended, and worked with some of the brightest and most courageous people who are working toward a cure and thriving with diabetes.

I am a journalist, writer, anchor, principal correspondent, and producer. I have reported from nearly every state in the United States, as well as from "hot zones" around the world: live fire, active wars, disaster areas on different continents, and even the watery catastrophe of New Orleans following Hurricane Katrina. I have received some of the highest awards in journalism and have interviewed presidents, an Oscar winner, supermodels, Nobel-caliber scientists, and world leaders.

I've done all that with an insulin pump or—before starting pump therapy—on a carefully measured regime of shots, testing my blood sugars, eating, re-testing my blood sugars, correcting, eating some more carbohydrates, and (yep, you guessed it) testing *yet again*.

I have made split-second decisions to travel down burned-out, blacked-out, blocked roads in post-earthquake Haiti, knowing that I was not near a hospital or any kind of immediate insulin supply if my personal supply got damaged or overheated; *knowing I was risking my life*, but also calmly knowing that I could do it because I had done it in the past. I knew that the people with whom I was working had my back and knew how to help if I got in trouble, and I knew that the risk was worth it and would enrich the lives of others.

I was nominated for a national *Emmy* award for knowing how to safely take those risks. I met leaders of a nation (Haiti) mired in struggle but also achingly resilient, dignified, and optimistic despite precious little material resources, food, and basics such as infrastructure, healthcare, education, or a working political and judicial framework.

I was voted *Best Reporter* in the most competitive local news market in the country by readers of a Miami newspaper. I even received the oh-so-coveted *Best Hair on the Air* on South Florida TV, an extremely competitive and lasting award (wink, wink). And I've done it all with type 1 diabetes.

Living with diabetes opened up a fascinating world to me: a world which I am uniquely qualified to investigate and share with viewers and readers—because I live with diabetes second by second, minute by minute, hour by hour, day by day, month by month and year by year.

So far, for more than twenty years!

What started as a seemingly certain early death sentence has become a lifestyle that probably has made me healthier than I would have been without diabetes, and it has given me a platform and job that helps others. It's an overused word, and it seems a little corny as I write this, but diabetes has enriched me and given me a purpose.

With the luxury of hindsight, I recognize that it should have been clear that something was seriously wrong as I spent long afternoons and even full evenings at the fast food burger joint on Main Street in Middletown, CT. This burger place was just steps away from the campus of Wesleyan University—a school that I had worked hard to get into. It was a school that represented all that had eluded me while growing up: mainstream academic success; accomplishment; a place reserved for many of the "best and the brightest."

That's what Wesleyan meant to me. Hanging out at the fast food burger place because it boasted free iced-tea refills *wasn't* what I had envisioned. (Unbeknownst to me at that time, the iced tea was like "poison." I had no idea that my immune system had turned against itself and that my pancreas was rapidly losing function.) It started as a constant, lingering thirst; that's why the free refills near Wesleyan were so prized.

I transferred to Wesleyan in the early 1990s from a college in the Midwest, following my older sister to the university where she had enjoyed a great academic run and was a standout student athlete. I wanted to be part of the Schmidt family tradition of academic excellence, and going to a school with sterling credentials and rigorous entrance requirements was a big part of that.

Yet after the elation of getting in wore off, and I began settling into the small campus along the Connecticut River in New England, things started to happen that felt increasingly strange and that just added to a near-constant sense of dread and anxiety.

Why now?

This was supposed to be a time of triumph and excitement, yet I couldn't make even basic decisions: where to live, what to study, whom to choose as an advisor, what to eat, whether I was too old (as a transfer student) to engage in the partying that other students enjoyed. I felt like an impostor and started having trouble keeping up with reading, getting out of bed, being "normal" or relaxed in my own skin and around students and faculty who welcomed me to the Wesleyan community.

I was painfully self-involved, anxious, and above all, *tired*. I was dragging, and what was worse, I was acutely aware of it as it was going on. While I should have been settling in, I developed a walloping sense of dread, lethargy, and helplessness. It was a painful and acute crisis of self-confidence. Maybe I really wasn't up to the challenges of a little Ivy League School? As I tried to adjust to my first semester at Wesleyan, I was met with a chorus of, "Why can't Benno just concentrate? If Benno would only focus, he'd do great." and repeated designations as a spectacular "underachiever." As I tried to get up to speed and into the most basic of college rhythms at Wesleyan, I just couldn't.

No sooner had I settled into my townhouse with other students that my comparisons to them started driving me crazy: *"How come I feel so awkward and obtuse, clumsy and deliberate?"* I would ask myself.

I didn't realize that my fascination with the local fast food burger place was really about my ever-increasing thirst. I lugged tons of books in my strained backpack on the often freezing walk to the burger place from Wesleyan. I was thirsty, and the burger place seemed like a good place to try and get some work done—even if I really didn't do much there other than stare at my books, wonder why I wasn't making progress, and stress out about assignments past due. All the while, I was enjoying those wonderful refills of iced tea.

I couldn't go anywhere without a cool drink, and my closest family members even had a term for it: "Benny is on *liquid patrol*"—as I raided their refrigerators for apple juice, diet soda, regular soda, or whatever was available to drink. I generally passed on milk, but my uncle and aunt even created a *liquid patrol* theme song as I stormed their house trying to quench my endless thirst.

Yet no matter how much I drank, I couldn't stop….

The studies were also beyond me, this after doing so well the previous semester. I often wondered, *"What the heck is wrong with me?"*

Professors were nice and patient and told me to come by anytime with specific questions about assignments or tests that they could address during office hours, but that was part of the problem: *I didn't have specific questions….*

Imagine a haggard, shockingly thin student barging into your office and bombarding you with basic, essential questions like…

"What's wrong with me?"

"How come I can't eat anything, have no appetite, and am thirsty all the time?"

They would look at me and suggest that I head over to the Student Health Center.

I didn't really want to go to the Health Center because that seemed like a colossal waste of time and effort. The *real* issue was reading assignments; I needed to concentrate. This was what I had wanted my entire high school life—just to be at a place like Wesleyan and feel that I belonged. I desperately wanted the academic success that was so flush in my family to include me too. I knew *something* was amiss, just not *what*.

I started making a lot of noise with anyone who would listen: friends, family, those same professors who were losing me in classes, my adviser, tennis partners—anyone patient enough to listen. This was my routine during those early months at Wesleyan: if you would stop and listen, I would share. My family was getting tired of the calls and questions. It was exhausting; their nephew, brother, son, cousin, friend and loved one was a "basket case."

My dad, whom I was named after, is a famous academic who led a university close to Wesleyan; he had finally had enough of my indecision. While I was visiting him, I asked him for the umpteenth time *that day* if I should stay or drop out of college. The indecision of this hyper-anxious young man was exasperating, and I didn't blame him or feel angry after his final reaction:

"It doesn't matter," he thundered, "which school you go to or even if you stay in school. What matters is that you do well at whatever choice you make and just let it unfold. This constant vacillating, this endless perseverating… it's…it's WORSE than crazy. It's b-o-r-i-n-g!"

Here is the reveal: My dad wasn't just an academic, and he didn't just lead a little university down the road a ways from Wesleyan. He is Benno C. Schmidt Jr., the former law clerk to Chief Justice Earl Warren while the court tackled the defining social issues of the last century. He's Benno C. Schmidt Jr., one of the youngest tenured faculty members in Columbia University's history before becoming its law school dean, all while still in his 30s. The same Benno C. Schmidt Jr. who became president of Yale University in his early forties, after Bartlett Giamatti left the Yale presidency to become a commissioner of major league baseball.

Another reveal: There's a valid reason that no one suspected a physical cause that first semester at Wesleyan. My mother, a beautiful, bright, accomplished artist and deeply caring hands-on parent, inherited a mental ailment to which she *never* surrendered. Like many others in her family, including her father (a celebrated New York City physician), my mom endured severe manic depression/bi-polar disorder for much of her adult life. She was there for my older sister and me, and she held together her own wonderful Greenwich Village apartment. She often managed her own life, but my mom also had sizeable episodes that required hospitalization and medication in an era when medications weren't as fine-tuned as they are now. I had seen her during many manic states, off of her medications, when her mood swings would take her to nonsensical, scary places.

As a student at Wesleyan—a student clearly falling apart—I always felt like an undefined entity: a kid who might have the smarts to do well academically like his father—or who might have inherited bi-polar disorder like his mother. I didn't know which was going to happen, and I wrongly thought that those two were my only choices. So those "what's wrong with me?" questions were really just shorthand for "do you think I am losing my mind?"

My mom was just about my age when her bi-polar disorder started affecting her. Was that what was going on here? Was I becoming bi-polar? Not a fair question to ask a professor, sister, father, drinking buddy, history instructor, or anybody, really, short of a psychiatrist armed with detailed blood work and my family history. I needed to see someone trained and extensively schooled in this stuff. Someone who could isolate traits and symptoms, who might, in fact, determine that something entirely different was to blame: a physical problem having little (and everything) to do with the frazzled mess I had become. Because of my mother's history of mental illness, others and I assumed that mental illness was to blame. The Health Center did too, after I came in with weight loss, depression, and anxiety—and certainly after I explained to the counselor that I had mental illness in my family.

My family believed it.

Liquid Patrol? Maybe that was simply a side effect of the anti-depressants you were on?

Weight loss and inability to concentrate?

Constant thirst?

How did it stop?

Where did it lead me—the weight loss, anxiety, inability to eat and concentrate, fear of losing my mind?

It wasn't to a locked mental hospital ward or padded cell somewhere....

It was, in the end, in my dorm room after my Uncle Bill Schmidt got one too many calls complaining of my depression. Uncle Bill finally said: "Something else may be going on here, and I'm going to investigate."

I spent a lot of time at his nearby home as my Wesleyan semester disintegrated. One day Uncle Bill came to my dorm to pick me up for a weekend, and he came a little early—thank God! He found me in bed—a skeleton really—down from 220 pounds to about 170 pounds and barely able to stand. After he took me home that Friday afternoon, he decided that the emergency room was a better fit. It didn't take the ER doctor long to diagnose me with full-blown, insulin-dependent type 1 diabetes. My dance, life, and journey with diabetes began.

Relief was all around. Family members were *happy* that I had diabetes, if you can imagine; it was a cause for my problems and persistent whining. I wasn't going crazy! I was simply dying from diabetes and needed insulin. I didn't need study sessions, office hours with professors, or anti-depressants.

I hadn't heard much about diabetes, except that you couldn't eat sugar and had to take shots. While unprepared, my entire family rallied and took up the cause. They learned about diabetes, and they collectively exhaled that *finally* they knew what was going on with Benny; he wasn't losing his mind—just his islet cells and insulin productivity!

What about now, as a middle-aged journalist who has lived really well with diabetes for over twenty years? My anxiety, depression, and attention problems didn't simply vanish with the diabetes diagnosis. They are still around and still cause some problems. I've learned, through my work with psychologists, that diabetes and depression are in fact linked, just not in the causal sense that I feared.

I used to hide or be ashamed of my diabetes; now I literally wear my diagnosis on my sleeve. I got a permanent medic alert bracelet tattooed on my inner right wrist that screams out *"Type 1 Diabetic"*—in case I ever get in trouble and a medic, paramedic, or doctor checks for a pulse on my inner wrist. Guess what? You can't lose your arm, and they will see the tattoo. I even shared that tattoo process with TV viewers worldwide, and the noted tattoo artist who *inked* me, Darren Brass, is himself living and thriving with diabetes. He's a bigger TV star than I, featured in the reality program *Miami Ink* for several seasons! We became friends over our love of living well with diabetes and our accepting and even enjoying the journey.

Diabetes hasn't held me back from going to Haiti numerous times before and after a devastating earthquake leveled the capital; having diabetes has even benefited my career in extraordinary ways.

Diabetes led to my hosting *dLife*, a program airing on CNBC and a website that is all about living well with diabetes, pursuing whatever dreams one has—again, all while living with this chronic condition. Thanks to *dLife*, the program I currently anchor, I've met extraordinary people living and thriving with diabetes. While on assignment for *dLife*, I've been involved with the most extensive, most involving, best-researched, best-told, and best-produced stories or segments available. *dLife* is seen online and on Sundays on CNBC at 7 p.m. Eastern Standard Time. (For further information about *dLife*, please see the website at the conclusion of this chapter.)

Here's the stark truth: No matter how good I may be at broadcast journalism, the founder of *dLife*—my mentor and friend Howard Steinberg—wasn't merely looking for just some pretty talking head who could write good cover stories about diabetes. There are plenty of those around who are desperate for interesting work in this evolving journalism climate. Howard wanted someone actually *living* with diabetes as he himself does; someone who has done well in his/her career while also managing and dealing with diabetes every second, every minute, every day, every week, every month, every year. This is where *dLife* and my diabetes have helped, broadened, even *sweetened* my life as a reporter. It wouldn't have happened without *dLife* and my living with diabetes.

While on assignment for *dLife*, I met Dr. Beverly S. Adler, the clinical psychologist and Certified Diabetes Educator whose life's work is helping others navigate diabetes and overcome depression and other emotional issues—setbacks that diabetes can and *does* bring. Howard, recognizing how deep the interplay of depression and diabetes is, bravely suggested a story for *dLife* that would feature Dr. Adler; she would bring this interplay to life for *dLife* viewers and website visitors.

I say *bravely* because, as topics for television broadcast, diabetes and depression are about as far as possible from the staples that drive local and network news to high ratings. Upon meeting "Dr. Bev," as she is called, I didn't immediately tell her about my diabetes history or my mom's struggles with severe bi-polar depression. The segment wasn't about me, nor was my history relevant. But since then, we've talked, and Dr. Bev knows how valuable and important I feel her work and mission are.

For our original *dLife* segment, Dr. Bev granted our team complete access to her Long Island office—even allowing us to document her session with a courageous patient confronting diabetes and the patient's dance with depression. For a journalist, this was *beyond* extraordinary. Forget about patient confidentially issues for a second. Consider what we (*dLife*) were allowed to document: a doctor and her patient tackling their most private, most challenging, most personal, and most potent hurdle—while doing it with a full production team of lights, cameras, and crew.

That is just *part* of what being a journalist with type 1 diabetes has allowed me to do. Those dark days in Middletown, CT over two decades ago turned into something challenging, annoying, maddening, and often exhausting, but they also morphed into a deeply rewarding, unexpected career niche. I've done plenty of political, cultural, social, sporting, or lifestyle segments and reports. They are fun, they get me out of my head, I enjoy them, and I do them well—competently and quickly. But none of them gets my journalism juices and mind engaged like stories concerning diabetes—none of them, regardless of the dateline, subject, or VIP whom I am interviewing.

I've benefited from the best treatment, the best minds, and the best training at the Diabetes Research Institute in South Florida. I have complete and total family support, the most understanding and loving wife that a person living with diabetes could have. I've also had fairly hassle-free access to test strips, insulins of all varieties and potencies, and insulin shot therapy with longer acting insulins and pump-therapy. I've even experimented with a continuous glucose monitor (CGM).

I now know that there is *nothing* wrong with me. It has been a colorful and upbeat journey. I can appreciate that I am someone who knows what diabetes is all about—not as a mere journalist and observer but as a member of the tribe. My father's words—*"What matters is that you do well at whatever choice you make"*—have guided my success. I've been to some extraordinary "hot zones" as a broadcast journalist, and while I won't say that doing all that as an insulin-dependent person with diabetes wasn't more challenging than for those without diabetes, it also hasn't held me back at all. In places like the Israeli border with Lebanon, or New Orleans after hurricane Katrina, I tell producers and photojournalists what diabetes is all about. I feel enormous pride and joy working for *dLife* and learning, researching, and reporting about a condition that nearly ended my life early many years ago.

One of the most inspirational quotes that I live by was spoken by Chris Waddell, a grade school classmate who was paralyzed in a ski accident. He rose to become one of the most decorated Olympians in U.S. History and even climbed Mt. Kilimanjaro in a wheelchair that he helped to design. His words were, "It's not what happens to you; it's what you do with what happens to you." My triumphs are the most powerful and lasting evidence that I can offer of that ongoing and rewarding life with diabetes.

www.dLife.com

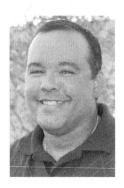

CHAPTER 21   *by George Simmons*

From Naive to Ninjabetic

"I would rather die than have to take shots for the rest of my life."
The words did not come out of my mouth, but I remember hearing them in my head. We were living with my grandparents when I was a kid, and one time I was watching my grandfather giving my grandmother a shot. She had type 2 diabetes, but at the time I didn't really understand diabetes at all. My grandma hated to take shots, so she made my grandpa give them to her. I remember how much she hated it, and seeing her face wince in pain, I knew that if I ever met that fate, I would rather end it all. The next year I watched my grandmother deteriorate and my grandfather do all that he could to take care of her. When she died in May of my eighth-grade year, it took my grandfather only six months to the day to join her. I guess, sometimes, it is hard to go on when your reason to live is gone.

Marching band was my outlet in high school. I went from just a plain old band member during my freshman year to drum section leader my sophomore year, to captain my junior year, and to drum major my senior year. Every Monday night, we had percussion rehearsal at school. It was my senior year and we were preparing for our first parade of the season. Rehearsal was going as planned when, all of a sudden, my band director asked me, "Are you feeling okay? You look pale." Being of both Cuban and Puerto Rican descent means that I am pretty dark skinned. Having someone describe me as "looking pale" was cause for concern.

"Well I feel a little light headed, but I am all right." Looking back, I remember that the feeling of light headedness became my normal. I figured that it was probably because I was up using the bathroom all night and not getting enough solid sleep. My mom came to band practice and took me to Urgent Care. That was the night that I was diagnosed with type 1 diabetes.

Sure, I had lost a lot of weight, but I assumed that it was due to all the exercise I was getting. Of course I was urinating all the time, I was thirsty all the time. All high school kids have mood swings. But I had lost too much weight. I looked awful. I was thirsty all the time, but no amount of water would ever satisfy me. And I always had been a pretty happy guy until recently, when my mother swore that I was like a different person.

There were so many warnings, but none that we recognized. And now I would have to take shots for the rest of my life. That night, the memory I had of that time at my grandparents' home popped into my head again. Did I tempt fate? Was I really going to choose dying over shots? Why did this happen to me?

When the time came, there was no question of what I was going to do. Of course I was going to choose life. Before we are put in a situation like that, it is easy to say the things that we sometimes say.

The next morning, we were to come back into the doctor's office for a blood draw and a shot of insulin. My doctor had me come back that afternoon for another blood draw to see how I was doing. All week long, I went in for blood draws both morning and afternoon. By the third day my arms were black and blue, so my nurse started drawing blood from my hands.

A nurse came to my house to teach me how to give myself shots. Since I was seventeen, I would have to learn all this stuff myself. My mother, although present, was not like some of the parents I had met. She stood back and let me take the driver's seat, since she knew I would be leaving the nest soon.

Taking that first shot must have taken me an hour. Holding that syringe and staring at the tip of the needle frightened me to no end, but the nurse was very understanding and reassuring, and that helped me to finally plunge that syringe into my thigh. It was a big deal to accomplish something I never thought I could do. It was the first triumph I had, in regards to my diabetes, that made me think I could actually handle this.

There was a class at a local hospital called "Understanding Diabetes" that my doctor suggested we attend. My mom called and got us a spot in the class. When I walked in, the first thing I realized was that I was the youngest person in the room. Next youngest was probably the teacher, then my mom, then all the rest of the people in the room. The instructor talked about watching the number of calories we would consume each day, but she stopped to say, "Not now for you, George. We need you to gain some weight." She said we needed to be careful with the amount of juice we would drink with breakfast, but she said, "Not now for you, George. You cannot drink juice anymore unless you are using it to treat low blood sugar."

The only things that I remember hearing that actually applied to me were that I should not drink juice, I should stay away from sweets like dessert, and I should not eat ketchup because there was a lot of sugar in ketchup. On and on, the instructor would say things to the group and then tell me how it didn't apply to me! I felt alone, isolated, annoyed, scared, frustrated, and just plain out of place. I was happy to leave that class, but still felt so much in the dark about diabetes.

Luckily I had a pretty good attitude about it all and knew that I had the rare kind of diabetes, unlike that of my late grandmother and those in the class. I was going to be fine.

Only a few weeks after my diagnosis, I received a call from a familiar voice.

"Hey George, how are you doing?" It was the Air Force recruiter from school whom I had been talking to about joining after graduation.

"I am doing okay. But I guess I do have some bad news." My story about being diagnosed and feeling like a total pincushion was easy to share. I remember feeling pretty good about being able to cry and to talk to him. That faith in myself and in my ability to overcome this disease was really strong at that time.

Then I noticed that he wasn't saying anything.

I waited.

"Wow, George." The disappointment in his voice was far worse than I expected. I was going to be fine, so what was the big deal? "I have some unfortunate news. The Air Force does not recruit people with diabetes. In fact, not any of the armed forces do. I am sorry, Son."

He heard the tears being held back as I said goodbye, but what he didn't know was how that moment would shape my attitude about diabetes. Diabetes just took away my future, in one phone call, and now what was I going to do?

Mom and Dad split when I was seven, but my father was always a part of my life. Having three sisters and a single mom meant that money was tight. My plan to join the Air Force had been fueled not only by my desire to serve my country, but by the need for an education that I could not afford on my own. I knew that the Air Force would enable me to both serve and go to school: a win-win if I had ever heard one. But now what was I going to do?

After high school, I got a job at a video store and was actually doing pretty well. Diabetes was just something that I knew I had but didn't really pay much attention to. I checked my blood sugar once or twice a day and continued taking my two prescribed shots every day, but that was it. I didn't think much about what I ate except that I stayed away from anything with sugar in it and did not drink juice.

One night when I was at work, I got a call from my mother. "Honey, I need you to come home and help me out. I am having some trouble with the car, and I need your help."

"Mom, I don't think I can leave, and I don't have a ride anyway. You should call someone else since I know nothing about cars." That was so weird. My brother-in-law was a mechanic; why would she want me to help?

"I already have arranged a ride for you and talked to your boss. I need you at home." She sounded so frustrated and at the same time drained. I hung up and waited for her friend to pick me up.

When I got home, I saw my sisters' cars parked out front and knew something was wrong. Walking into the living room and seeing no one but my stepfather was confusing. He directed me into my mom's bedroom. Sitting around her bed were my sisters and my brother-in-law. Mom told me as well as she could that my dad had had a heart attack that morning while he was on vacation in Arizona with my stepmom. Before I could ask how he was, Mom told me that he had died instantly.

My fists hurt from punching the wall, and my throat hurt from wailing in sorrow. I remember wondering how many tears any one person could produce. The pain and emptiness that I felt were immense. It was just over a year after I was diagnosed, and my father was gone. How would I deal with all this? My future was taken away by diabetes, and now my father was gone? How could I go on? What was I going to do?

Divorce was not pretty. I am sure that, in some instances, couples are civil to one another for their kids' sake, but that was not the case with my parents. My mom and dad would have us kids deliver messages to one another, because any time they spoke, their conversation ended in an argument. That night, after I calmed down, my mother told me a story that really blew my mind.

"You know what is weird? Last night your Dad called here. He was looking for you. He asked if you were home, but I told him that you were working. I was ready to hang up, but then he asked about you. He said he had been worried about you and your diabetes and wanted to check on you."

"The funny thing was that we talked for a long time. I mean like almost two hours. We talked about each one of you kids, how proud we are of all of you, and about lots of good times we had together. He brought up stuff we did when we were dating, and we laughed and laughed. There were so many great memories that I had not thought about in a long time. It reminded me of why I first fell in love with him."

"It's like he knew. Or that God decided to clear things up with us before he died. Anyway, I wanted you to know." She couldn't talk anymore, and I didn't need to hear anything else. We hugged and cried. I sobbed some more as she held me and rubbed my back.

The conversation that they had really was a gift to us kids. Going to our mother for comfort with Dad's death was difficult since most of the memories we had were of them arguing. But that phone call made it okay. In a weird way, it almost erased the memories of all of those fights.

Going on after that was tough. The pain and emptiness that I felt led to some pretty deep depression. I could tell that my health suffered from it, since every time I checked my blood sugar, it was in the 200s mg/dL.

Although I continued to take my insulin as prescribed, I checked my blood sugar less and less often and would go to the doctor only when he refused to refill my prescriptions. I was a mess, and to top it all off, I started drinking alcohol, smoking, and doing drugs.

The way that I dealt with it all was to numb myself every night, so I could sleep and to smoke all day to hurt myself. I would never remember going to sleep at night, but I would wake up with empty bottles of alcohol on my dresser, the lights still on, and my head pounding. A few years later, I stopped the drinking and drugs, knowing that I needed to pull my life together. I started dating a woman whom I used to date in high school, and we got very serious very early on. She remembered when I was diagnosed, back in high school, since she was in marching band too. But because I hadn't mentioned it much, she had never asked me about it.

Fast forward to fourteen years later. Now we are married, have two kids, and are just getting by as most young couples do. Life really turned around for me when I started going to church, and my faith really filled that void in my heart. I still did not worry much about diabetes, and miraculously, I had no major issues.

One day I got sick. I was at work and felt awful. I knew that a few people in the office had battled the stomach flu, so I assumed that flu was the issue. After barely making it to the bathroom to vomit, I knew I had to go home. I called my wife and headed out. I was only a few miles away from my home when I felt like I would throw up again. I didn't know what to do. I was dripping in sweat, and there was no way I could make it home.

The local grocery store was right near me, so I pulled into the parking lot and parked very close to the street so that I could avoid the people coming out of the store. I got out of my car and into the back seat, where I used a paper bag that I found on the floor. People were walking by, and I just kept vomiting over and over. I thought I would never stop. It was terrifying.

After my stomach finally calmed, I grabbed my cell phone and told my wife what had happened. I felt a lot better and took off, hoping to make it home without another pit stop. When I got home, my wife wanted to get something in me since dry heaves are so painful. Having kids taught me all about the

"B.R.A.T. diet": Bananas, Rice, Applesauce, and Toast were the best foods for someone with nausea. The thought of anything made me feel ill, so I just went to bed.

My wife asked, "What about your shot?"

"I cannot keep anything down," I told her. "If I take a shot, my blood sugar will go too low."

Back then, I really thought that was the case. No one had ever told me that you need insulin just for your body to work. I thought it was all about balancing food intake. So my brain thought that, without the ability to keep food in me, I should not take any insulin.

Lying in bed, I felt weak and dizzy. My eyes closed as the room spun, and I fell asleep. I am not sure how long I slept, but I woke up feeling sick again. My wife had left a glass of water on my nightstand. I took a sip of water to try and quench my thirst and almost instantly felt it coming back up. Stumbling to the bathroom alerted my wife to my state. She saw me lying there on the floor not able to keep anything down and demanded that I check my blood sugar.

She grabbed my dusty machine and handed me the lancing device. She stuck the strip in the machine, and I pricked my finger. She lowered the machine to the droplet of blood on my finger and said, "This just says 'High.' What does that mean? How high?"

I told her that I believed it meant that I was *over* 600 mg/dL. We checked again, and it was the same. Not knowing what to do, I asked her to bring me a syringe and my bottle of Regular insulin. I took twenty units into my thigh and sat there on the floor wondering just how high I was and why. My wife decided to call 911, so I tried to get to the family room near the back door where they would probably park. I barely made it halfway there and ended up on the couch in our living room.

Flashes of scenes come to mind: Two EMTs standing over me; our neighbor talking to my wife outside the ambulance; the ceiling of the ambulance; the blue sky twisting from left to right and quickly disappearing into a constant flow of fluorescent lights. One after another, they passed like the lines painted on a highway.

When I was admitted to the emergency room, they did another blood sugar test from my finger, and their machine also just said "High." How high did I get? It must have been over forty minutes since I had taken that shot, right? Was this the same day? How long have I been here?

I spent the next few days in ICU and then was moved into a regular room for a day or two. A doctor came in to see me one afternoon and explained that I needed insulin no matter what. I felt like an idiot.

"Actually, we get a lot of people in DKA who don't understand how it all works." He explained that DKA stood for *diabetic ketoacidosis*—a problem that occurs in people with diabetes when the body cannot use sugar (glucose) as a fuel source because there is no insulin or not enough insulin to convert that glucose into energy. Fat is used for fuel instead, which creates a byproduct called *ketones*. A high level of *ketones* causes the blood to become acidic, like poison, which can be fatal. He made it clear that my poor education and lack of understanding could have kept me out of the hospital. It made me realize that I needed to seek out the knowledge that I lacked. I was determined to get my diabetes life together.

The doctor suggested that I see an endocrinologist. For fifteen years, I had had diabetes and had never seen an endocrinologist. I didn't know what an endocrinologist was! Luckily, I was referred to a great endocrinologist in my area and saw him soon after. He spent a lot of time explaining to me that I was really in control of my disease. Daily shots cannot be considered just a static standard dose since my blood sugar level, activity, food intake, and exercise can alter my insulin needs.

We discussed sliding scales and procedures for properly taking shots. He explained that I should be checking my blood at least eight times a day: once when I wake up, before every meal, two hours after every meal, and before bed. I hadn't been checking for months, and now I would be checking eight times a day? That was all new to me, but I was ready and willing.

That appointment was overwhelming, but so informative. I had no idea what an A1c was, let alone what mine was. There were so many things that I never knew. It made me wonder how many more people out in the world did not understand diabetes.

I had recently purchased an iPod and loved listening to it all the time. Podcasts were a new part of the iTunes store, and I had just discovered them. Podcasts are just audio shows, like talk radio, except not live. You can subscribe to the shows you like and every time you sync your iPod to your computer, new episodes would automatically be downloaded to it for listening.

A quick search for "diabetes" in the iTunes store pulled up a podcast called *DiabeticFeed*. I double clicked on the first episode and waited in anticipation while it loaded. When I heard the host say that she was a person living with type 1 diabetes and would report during each episode on diabetes news in the world, I knew that it would quickly become my favorite show. Each week I would listen as soon as a new show was added. One week, she had a guest on the show, a diabetes blogger named Kerri Morrone who had type 1 diabetes and had decided to share her diabetes life online to help connect with others.

Blogging was not something I had ever done, nor did I read any blogs. But now I had to check it out. What I found changed my life forever and for the better. That blog led me to other blogs, and I quickly started corresponding and reaching out to these other people with type 1 like me! I had never met another person with type 1 diabetes, so this was the first time that I felt "normal."

When you live with diabetes, it is hard to feel normal.

People with diabetes have to make themselves bleed several times day. Some have to draw up syringes with insulin and give themselves shots. They have to see the numbers on their blood glucose machines and know what to do with them. They have to count carbohydrates in the food they eat, remember to refill prescriptions, make and attend doctors' appointments, exercise, check their feet, and listen to their bodies for any changes like *hypoglycemia* (low blood sugar). People with diabetes are like super humans.

When I was a kid, I thought ninjas were the coolest. They could climb anything, hide anywhere, and sneak up on you without a sound. Like super humans! Which is why, when I decided to start my own blog, I called it, "Ninjabetic," with the tagline, "Because it takes being a ninja to live successfully with diabetes." And frankly, I believe that is the case. (For further information about my "Ninjabetic" blog, please see the website at the conclusion of this chapter.)

Almost every day, I would write a little something about my life: doctors' appointments, frustrations, failures, successes, and everything in-between. People started to read it and to comment on posts that I had written. A dialog would begin around a post, and more relationships would form with each comment. I now had lots of friends with type 1 diabetes, like me.

The fact is that we are not meant to go it alone. We need each other. As soon as I was connected to this Diabetes Online Community (DOC), I knew that I was going to be okay. Having a community to share with, learn from, and feel a part of changed my attitude about diabetes. It made me want to take better care of myself.

At that time I was still taking multiple daily injections of insulin. It was working pretty well, but I was struggling to get my morning blood sugar levels down. It seemed that, no matter what I did at night, I would still end up with a higher than desired blood sugar number each morning. Since I was so frustrated about this issue, I decided to write a blog post about it. It wasn't long before several of my friends suggested that I look into an insulin pump. I had heard about them, but never thought I wanted one. The thought of having a device stuck to me all day long seemed awful. But after hearing so many positive comments, I decided to ask my doctor about it.

At my next appointment I talked with him about the pros and cons of using an insulin pump. He explained that many people with type 1 diabetes were finding a lot of freedom and tighter control using insulin pumps. We talked about the morning blood sugar highs and how the insulin pump would enable me to turn up my insulin delivery in the early morning to help eliminate the spike that would occur each day. I was sold. A few weeks later, I found myself at an Introduction to Insulin Pumping class.

My wife attended the meeting with me for support and for her own education. After seeing how much more involved and focused I was about my diabetes, it made her want to learn more too. During the class, the instructor handed each of the people with diabetes a pump to look at and told us that in a few minutes we would all put on an infusion set and pump saline during the class. I will admit that I was kind of scared at the thought of trying a pump for the first time in front of all those people. The instructor asked if anyone of the people who came to the class wanted to try a pump too. Those of us with diabetes laughed and looked around the room to see if any of our spouses, significant others, or family members who came with us would try it.

"I'll try it!" The voice sounded as though it came from right next to me. It turned out to be my wife—the only person in the room without diabetes who was willing to try wearing a pump! I was so very proud of her and felt pretty lucky to have such awesome support from my spouse.

I now use insulin pump therapy to manage my diabetes, and I love it. Does it have some negative issues that come along with it? Sure. I get annoyed sometimes at the tubing that runs from the pump to the infusion site on my body. Sometimes it can get caught on things like doorknobs or dresser drawer handles, which can not only hurt if ripped out but can also be really frustrating if I have to stop and put in a new infusion set. Still, I would not go back to daily insulin injections. I really love the pump.

Now that I was using an insulin pump and checking my blood sugar ten to twelve times a day, I knew that I needed to take on something that I had been ignoring for a long time. To say that I was going to take better care of myself and yet to not quit smoking was a complete contradiction. Drinking and drugs were no longer a part of my life and had not been for a long time, but I still smoked. I smoked a pack of cigarettes every day for over fifteen years, and although I did try to quit many times, it never seemed to stick.

Now I knew that I had many people cheering me on who would also hold me accountable. I needed that accountability. So I picked a date, bought nicotine patches, and wrote a post about it. I let it all out, and my friends online all encouraged me to quit. They were there for me every step of the way, and I have not had a cigarette since. It has been over five years now, and I can say wholeheartedly that I am a non-smoker. Frankly it is hard to imagine that I ever did smoke.

Never would I have thought that a bunch of people typing messages to me on a computer could help me take better care of myself. Never did I think that I would count so much on their support. But I do. It is my new normal. My community.

The next few months were wild. Emails came flooding into my inbox, telling me how I inspired others to quit smoking too. Some people who had smoked even longer than I had decided that if I could do it, they could too! It was amazing. My life was affecting others in a positive way and that was something I always hoped would happen but never knew how. What an awesome feeling to know that I was helping to change people's lives.

One thing that was still missing for me was actually meeting someone face to face with type 1 diabetes. I knew lots of people online, but no one locally. Then I had the good fortune to meet many of my online friends for dinner or coffee when they came into town. It was, is, and will always be something that I continue to do. Giving a real hug to these people with whom I share so much of life is the best!

My daughter had a good friend from school who was also on her soccer team. We had met the little girl's parents and had quickly become good friends with them. On the first day of school, we got a call from her mom. She informed us that their youngest daughter, who was just going to start Kindergarten that day, ended up in the hospital and was diagnosed with type 1 diabetes.

My heart broke. I assured them that, if they needed any help or anything at all, to please give us a call. I called the local JDRF chapter (formerly known as the Juvenile Diabetes Research Foundation) and asked about their programs for newly diagnosed families. They gave me information, phone numbers, and email addresses of people who could be there for the family. I was glad that they reached out, but at the same time I wished I could do more.

I shared all that I learned with the family and also told them about blogs by other parents of children with diabetes. They were thankful and found a lot of comfort reading those blogs and reaching out to those parents. Once again, togetherness and the Diabetes Online Community provided some hope and comfort.

When you feel as though you are all alone, it is easy to get scared. I remember that, as a kid, I always wanted to go to bed before everyone else. Just knowing that someone was awake in the house helped me go to sleep. Surely they would watch out for me and alert me if anything was wrong. People in your corner; people who care.

Something I hear myself say often is that this Diabetes Online Community saved my life. I mean that literally. Sure, it was that incident with DKA that started this journey, but the community that I found online gave me the encouragement I needed to continue down the path to good health.

I think back to my Grandma and how much she hated having diabetes. I think about how so many of my family have and still struggle with type 2 diabetes. The prevalence of type 2 diabetes in the Latino community is staggering and growing at alarming rates. How many of those people need community? My guess is that many of them feel alone. I would imagine there are several who feel as my Grandma did. As I did.

Maybe there are people on this earth who can keep themselves motivated all the time. Maybe there are people who never get down when things get tough:

people who don't ever get tired of doing the same thing over and over, and who never feel as though they want to give up. I am sure those people exist, but I don't know anyone like that, and I am definitely not like that.

Every few months, I feel depressed. I may struggle, but I never feel alone. When I feel down, I reach out to the online community, to my friends, and they are always there for me with an encouraging word, an inspiring message, or even a phone call if needed. I am never alone, and with that, I know that I will be able to get through anything that diabetes decides to throw my way. The power of community holds me up and keeps me going.

I was recently asked what advice I would give to someone who was newly diagnosed with diabetes. I said, "Find a community and stay connected." Isolation can be paralyzing, but it is also completely unnecessary. There might not be people around the corner from you, but there are people who can and will be there for you, if you just reach out and stay connected to a community.

It can change your life.

www.ninjabetic.com

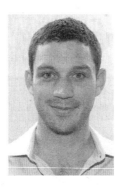

CHAPTER 22   *by John Sjölund*

Diabetes: Always Something There to Remind Me...

I had been training for this race for over six months. I had spent hours and hours on the rowing machine at my gym while I was at university in Jönköping, Sweden. Then I rolled around on roller skis while working as an intern at a human resources consulting firm in Singapore. As if being six-foot three-inches tall wasn't enough to make me stick out in Asia, here I was on funny-looking skis with wheels in the 90°F heat of Singapore. I also stuck out as I practiced going up hills at a golf course in Stockholm, Sweden. Having grown up while my father trained for—and ultimately completed twenty-three times—the longest cross-country ski race in the world, it was my turn to participate in *Vasaloppet*, held on the first Sunday of March every year. The world's oldest and—in popular consideration, the biggest—cross-country ski race, *Vasaloppet* is an annual long-distance (90-km/56-mile) event that takes place in northwestern Sweden between the towns of *Sälen* and *Mora*.

Now you might think that every Swede is born on skis and grows up skiing ten miles in the snow every day to school and back. Not the case for this Swede. I grew up in Connecticut in a suburb outside of New York City, and cross-country skiing was not my main mode of transport! Besides not really knowing how to ski prior to setting off on this challenge to complete *Vasaloppet*, I had been living with type 1 diabetes since the age of three and had never before completed an endurance race. I was entering new territory in managing my diabetes, but at age twenty-one, I was determined to study the balance between carbohydrates, exercise, and insulin—all while figuring out how to stay up on my two feet on thin cross-country skis. This endeavor was the result of a family friend who, while we were lunching on pasta and diet cokes, dared me to do the race with him.

I was diagnosed with diabetes one week before my fourth birthday. To me, it seems that I have lived with diabetes my entire life. This condition (I hate it when people call it a disease!) has never defined who I am, but it certainly has played a large part in my life, even becoming my full-time career. The day I was diagnosed with diabetes doesn't feature centrally in my memory, but a picture of the day, taken by my dad, does take up center stage in the photo album of my early years. In the picture, I am sitting in a narrow hospital bed with a giant smile on my face. Of course the smile wasn't a result of being diagnosed, or of having an intravenous drip hooked up to my arm, but rather was due to a gift my parents had given me; I think it was some kind of car-racing set. My smile is as big today, twenty-six years later, as it was in the Children's Ward at Greenwich Hospital on that Friday in May 1986.

Would I choose to live with diabetes if I didn't have to? Definitely not. But there are many, many problems in this world that I would much rather solve before curing my own diabetes. Sometimes I have good diabetes days, and sometimes they are bad. There is nothing more frustrating than—when the pressure is on, a deadline is looming—my blood sugar goes bouncing from *hypoglycemic* (low blood sugar) to *hyperglycemic* (high blood sugar) and back to *hypoglycemic* as I overcompensate. Generally, I just try to get on with life and take care of my diabetes in the best possible way. There are too many places to visit, too many people to meet, and too many things to learn to let me get dragged down by a non-functioning pancreas!

I often get asked what it is like to live with diabetes. The closest comparison I have come up with is that it's like having a humming in your ear all the time—perhaps something like tinnitus. Sometimes it is very soft, sometimes louder, but there is something in your system that you need to be in tune with, and it cannot be ignored for more than a short period of time. It is as if we people living with diabetes have an extra internal dialogue that needs to be dealt with.

> *"Why am I so thirsty? Why do the muscles in my arm feel a little sore? How many carbohydrates are in a ramen noodle dish? Why did I wake up an extra hour early this morning? Why am I having a tough time concentrating on this legal document that I should be reading? Why am I getting beads of sweat on my forehead? I just urinated a few minutes ago—why do I need to go again? Why is my hand shaking? Why am I getting irritated at my lovely and patient wife for no reason? Do I have my insulin with me? When did I take my last injection? Did I double dose? Oh no! I just double dosed! What do I do now?"*

It's a full-time job constantly checking in with your body, but after twenty-six years, I struggle to imagine how people cannot do it! It has become a natural part of my life rhythm to do a little "wellness check" with my body every so often—and if you live with diabetes, you'll realize that this little check occurs every couple of minutes.

…67, 66, 65, 64 kilometers to go, and things are going okay. The wax on my skis was giving me the right combination of grip to get the speed and glide to propel me forward. It was an amazing Sunday, the culmination of six months of training, and I was fulfilling what I thought was an impossible dream: me, someone with type 1 diabetes, aiming to complete the *Vasaloppet* race with my father, who was sixty-three years old at the time.

33, 32, 31…..26, 25….18, 17 going fine. 16, 15… here comes a big downhill. Finally, I can go into a tuck and rest my poor body. *"Why did I do this again??"* … SPLAT! Face first into the snow, skis spread behind me, one ski pole facing up the hill, and literally thousands of skiers coming past me in this downhill section of the race. I had completed seventy-five kilometers of *Vasaloppet* and had only fifteen kilometers to the finish line when a momentary lack of concentration caused me to collapse in the middle of the ski course, legs burning, close to exhaustion, wondering how on earth I would get up from this and keep going. I maneuvered myself off to the side, stood up on one leg, took a little break, wondered if I could blame this fall on my diabetes (I couldn't, that came later), got up on the other leg, zig-zagged up to get my pole. Reset, started to ski again. *"What did I get myself into…?"*

I'm a guy who likes to work towards goals that I set for myself, both professionally and personally. My wife calls these my "lists." They keep things organized and, with so many things on the go, they help me to keep track of the calls, emails, meetings, birthdays, memos, chats, movie titles, book titles, band names, potential races, and people whom I try to keep in the front of my mind. I just turned thirty, and a couple of days before my birthday, I sat down and made a list of things that feature most prominently in my life:

- I am married to an incredible woman from *Namibia*, whom I met while on a hike around the Cape of Good Hope (how fitting) while I was living in South Africa.
- My relationship with my family is one of the most important things in my life.
- I have lived in the U.S., Sweden, South Africa, Switzerland, Singapore, and the UK and travel regularly all over for fun and, more recently, in relation to my diabetes.
- I have friends scattered across the globe who love and support me unconditionally.

- I have completed a number of half marathons, triathlons, and both of the largest organized bike and cross-country ski races in the world.
- I volunteer my time to a fantastic program developed by the International Diabetes Federation (IDF) as part of the faculty for their Young Leaders Programme.
- I am co-founder and CEO of "Timesulin," a company that I passionately believe is making a difference in the lives of people with diabetes.
- I was recently recognized as one of the Ten Outstanding Young People (TOYP) in Sweden for medical innovation related to Timesulin—aiming to end the anxiety that some of us feel when not remembering if/when we took our last insulin injection.
- Oh, and I have lived with type 1 diabetes, myself, since I was four years old.

I am the youngest of three brothers, and my parents got the shock of their lives when I was diagnosed with type 1 diabetes. We were a Swedish family living in America, and no one in my family had ever lived with type 1 diabetes (or type 2, for that matter). My mother had recognized that I had to go to the bathroom much more often than normal, and off I went to the hospital to get it checked out. Diabetes. As odd as it may sound, I've never really known life without diabetes, and my childhood memories are so positive, that having this chronic condition has never featured prominently. I often get asked if the fact that I have had it my "whole" life has made it easier to manage. I have no doubt that it has made it easier for me to live such a fulfilling and balanced life with diabetes, but I think that it also has to be a question of attitude.

One of the greatest experiences—and what I credit as the biggest influence on my life as someone with diabetes, aside from my parents—were my summers spent at Camp Joslin, a summer camp outside of Boston, MA for kids with diabetes. I was a camper at Camp Joslin five years in a row between the ages of eight and thirteen, a critical age in transitioning from child to teenager. It's tough enough to make that transition for the average kid, but when you need to take extra responsibility for yourself and your diabetes, it can be an incredible challenge. Camp Joslin, I believe, got me through it in one piece. I remember so well a Swedish counselor who was on summer break and volunteering at Joslin during the first summer that I attended. (Stereotypically enough, his name was Sven, and he was a professional skier, if memory serves correctly.) Sven immediately picked up on the fact that I was new to summer camps and to this environment, and took me under his wing for the two weeks that I was there. To say that this Swedish guy—a professional skier—became a hero to eight-year-old me is an understatement. I think I decided that day that I would also become a professional skier. (Okay, I haven't made it yet, but perhaps completing *Vasaloppet* got me closer??) The amazing thing about Camp Joslin was that nearly everybody there—including kids, staff, nurses, administration, lifeguards, etc.—had diabetes themselves. It was the one place in the world where I was just another boy doing all the things that other boys did: quarter-mile swim competitions, fishing, soccer, arts and crafts, sailing, ghost stories around the camp fire. Every location around the camp was set up so that if anything diabetes-related happened—a low blood sugar, for example—it could be dealt with immediately, on the spot, and without being a big deal. Additionally, structured education was a key part of the camp. It felt like just another activity at the time, but we all got to learn the importance of regular exercise and how to manage our diabetes effectively, plan our meals, and maintain blood sugar control. All of a sudden, if everyone around you is talking about blood sugar, weighing food to learn how many grams of protein are in a chicken breast, eating snacks before swimming a quarter mile, drinking extra water when there is a risk of ketones—it just isn't a big deal anymore. I still think back fondly on the hall where we ate our meals at the Joslin Camp. I didn't think about it at the time, but today, to recall sitting in a room with 150 other people of all ages, all dealing with diabetes...what an amazing feeling. We are a community of people who are very different, but we have this one common element that unites us: Diabetes. And the most important thing for us to realize is that it is up to us to take care of our diabetes in the best possible way we can.

With all the positive memories I have of growing up, I'm the first one to admit that I had some serious diabetes wobbles in my teenage years. I was stubborn and in denial, and I refused to go to my doctor and test my blood sugar. In the end, I always succumbed and just got on with it. And for this, I honestly credit my parents for being supportive, loving me unconditionally, providing me with balance, and never judging. Life with diabetes is challenging, and we all slip up sometimes. I sure did. (And between you and me, I still sometimes do... we're human, after all!)

When I was fifteen years old, after finishing the ninth grade in Connecticut, I followed in the footsteps of my oldest brother and decided to head to Sweden to attend a boarding school called *Sigtunateskolan Humanistiska Läroverket*, or SSHL. I had a great time as a student there. That was the first time in my life that I was truly on my own to manage my diabetes. Thinking back, perhaps it was a little crazy, but I survived. I never looked at my diabetes as any sort of hindrance, but just got on with all things student-related. After finishing high school, I did something that is very common in Europe, but quite unusual in America: I took a "gap year."

The basic goal of the gap year was to have as much fun as possible, which I did. But everything leading up to the fun times, and everything following after the fun times, was anything but fun! In order to finance my goal of being a (working) ski bum, I did some research to determine the highest salary

I could earn with just a high school diploma. I started this journey as a substitute teacher in Stockholm. It was a great experience. I mentored and taught two Iraqi immigrant students for over a month; I taught a gym class at my cousin's school; and I was even a Spanish teacher for a week and a half, despite not being able to speak Spanish at all. It wasn't until my close friend, Kim, came up with a recommendation that I found the highest-paying job that did not require higher education—as a window washer! So from being a substitute teacher, I moved to offices all around Stockholm polishing windows. Because we got paid per surface that we cleaned, and with Swedish offices always having at least double glazing for insulation, we all started developing our own techniques for polishing as many windows as possible, as quickly as possible. One of my more memorable experiences was being assigned to a hospital in Stockholm called *Karolinska Sjukhus* for the entire summer. Basically, I walked from floor to floor and cleaned every single window, including the ones in the operating rooms, requiring me to put on full scrubs before entering. It was great to receive that hefty paycheck at the end of each week that summer and the one after; it was lucrative, and I was a money-hungry teenager! However, I distinctly remember how people looked down on me when I came in with the bucket and squeegee and treated me as if I were less worthy because of the job I had chosen. People were rude to me, made me feel as though I was inconveniencing them and wasting their time, when all I was trying to do was make their office a little cleaner and complete my own goals. I learned from that experience the true meaning of the phrase "treat others the way you want to be treated yourself." It was sad how poorly I was treated during that time, and it made a lasting impression on me. Despite my poor social standing, I achieved my goal: to follow my passion for snowboarding and move to the Swiss Alps for a winter season.

Getting back to my gap year and snowboarding, the destination of choice was *Verbier*, located in the French part of Switzerland. With my friends, Erik and Amanda, I rented a tiny house for the season and managed to find a job at a winter camp designed to accommodate large groups of kids who came on school trips to visit the Alps. But the job wasn't the important part here. The important part was that I was able to go snowboarding every single day, and I did. Those of us who ski or snowboard normally have only a couple of days per year in which to be outside enjoying the mountains and experiencing the thrill of skiing/ snowboarding. It also follows that, during that time, usually limited to a week's break, you try to ski every single day, regardless of the weather conditions. The beauty of *living* in the mountains for a few months was that I didn't need to feel guilty if I decided not to go skiing for a day. So what lesson did I learn from this entire experience? No combination of exercise, altitude, lack of supplies, or other diabetes-related challenge stopped me from having fun and doing what I wanted to do with my friends.

As much as I want to imagine that any success I have managed to achieve was due to my athletic prowess, sadly it wasn't. The real keys to any success that I have reached were the result of working hard, taking risks, relentlessly networking with my peers, and being open to experiencing new things. During my studies at the Jönköping International Business School, which focused on entrepreneurship and international studies, I went on an exchange year to Durban, South Africa. During that year, I fell in love with South Africa and eventually found a job that would allow me to stay in Cape Town for an extended period.

While I was finishing my Master's thesis about entrepreneurships in the townships of Cape Town, South Africa, I knew that this country was where I wanted to stay. For those of you who have had the chance to visit South Africa, and Cape Town in particular, you will probably recognize how amazing this place is. Located on the southern tip of Africa, it has great food, surfing, wine farms, and a huge mountain ("Table Mountain") in the middle of the city. It was pretty incredible! I was lucky enough to become acquainted with two Swedish entrepreneurs living in the city, and I was sold. I made it my goal to find a job that would allow me to live in Cape Town. Towards the end of my thesis research, my older brother was in Cape Town visiting. When I told him of my grand plans to try to stay in Cape Town, he remembered that he had a friend of a friend who was one of Africa's first users of *Skype*, the VOIP-calling software that my brother was involved in creating. After sending some emails, we were able to find the contact details of the president of an amazing company called Acceleration eMarketing. Acceleration worked within digital marketing to provide world-class digital marketing technology and services to companies around the world with outsourced services provided from their hub in Cape Town, which I wanted to join.

Now when I say "outsourcing," you're probably picturing not being able to communicate with the workforce because of linguistic barriers, cultural sensitivity, time zones, and bad phone connections. The beauty about Cape Town was its cultural similarity to Europe. Not only was Cape Town culturally similar, it didn't have the biggest companies in the world recruiting all of your best staff, as often happens in Silicon Valley. Therefore, the company could recruit and retain super smart people who were world leaders in their trades. I suppose it might have been a stroke of luck, since all I wanted was to find a way to stay in South Africa, but I ended up spending the next five years working at a wonderful company where I learned a ton about management, business, and relationships. I started as an email campaign manager responsible for the technology stack and deployment of commercial email messages (no spamming, I promise), and I was able to learn the trade in Cape Town. Along my path with Acceleration, I was transferred first to New York City to manage a section of their client base in North America and then over to London to build a new business area. This little company that I found by a stroke of luck, and got recruited to over a lunch in Cape Town, ended up being a fantastic place to gain skills and experience that would later enable me to fulfill my own dreams of starting a business of my own.

I recall a time when I was in Skype's London office presenting my suggestion for how to increase the conversion rates of their new-member emails, when the dreaded beads of sweat started forming on my forehead. This wasn't happening because I was nervous about giving this presentation (which I was, but that honestly wasn't causing me to sweat), but rather because I felt a *hypoglycemic reaction* coming on. So what did I do? Since I didn't have anything with me to treat my low blood sugar, I had to stop the meeting and rush out onto the street to the nearest shop where I could buy some candy. On returning, fearing the worst, I was met by an incredibly concerned group of people who wanted nothing more than to ensure that I was okay. They suggested that we cancel the entire meeting and re-schedule so that I could regroup. It wasn't necessary; I was happy to continue when my blood sugar returned to normal, and I was very impressed and glad to be working with such good people.

After just over five years working with Acceleration in South Africa, USA, and the UK, it finally was time to spread my wings and venture into the world of entrepreneurship. During my time at university, I had learned much of the theory about entrepreneurship, but it wasn't until I rolled up my sleeves and gave it a try that I really learned what it was about.

Having been a multi-day insulin pen injector for many years, I had a recurring problem that I never could seem to get past. I took insulin four or five times per day, every single day, which became a huge amount of insulin injections—roughly 1500 shots every year! Most of the time, all went well, but sometimes—at least once per week—I *forgot* if I had taken my injection or not. Typically, this anxious feeling of not remembering happens within a few minutes of when I thought I did (or did not) actually take it. I could be seated at the dinner table with my wife, still eating an appetizer, when the dreaded feeling would come back. Normally I tried to retrace the steps in my own head. *"Did I lift my shirt to expose my belly? Did I grab the pen out of my pocket/back/ jacket/ from the table? Did I put it back in the refrigerator in a certain place?"* Sometimes, I was able to successfully determine if I took it, sometimes not. If I couldn't remember, the next step would be to ask those people around me if they had seen me take my insulin. If we were eating dinner around a table, the answer was normally yes; however, people normally aren't around me when I take my insulin. The third and final tactic, which could be embarrassing to admit, was the Sniff Test. (I should really trademark this one...) Insulin has a strong and distinct smell to it. A short time after injecting, you can ask someone to smell your belly (if you are lucky) or your bottom, if you are unlucky (perhaps I should say if they are unlucky) to see if any insulin is left around the injection site. If the other person has a keen sense of smell, he or she might be able to confirm whether or not you had administered the shot. My point is this: that actual moment or two when I'm giving myself an insulin injection is largely unmemorable, but the risks of double dosing—or of skipping a dose—are dire.

Having had this problem for many years, I was always asking my doctors if there wasn't some smarter way to handle this. I often got one of two responses:

1. I have heard about big companies working on this product; it will come in the future. (It never has.)

2. How is it possible that you forget whether you have taken this life-sustaining medicine? Surely you should just try harder to remember.

Neither response was satisfactory to me.

From my own experiences, I knew that this issue of forgotten injections, and the associated worry that I would accidently take a double injection and risk a potentially severe *hypoglycemic reaction*, took a lot of energy. In addition to checking in with our body's physiological responses, testing blood sugar, counting carbohydrates, and remembering supplies, having to deal with forgotten insulin injections is yet another piece of baggage that we carry around with us every day, and I wanted to solve it. My attitude about most questions in life is that, if I have a question, problem, or concern, there is probably someone who has the same issue. Even though I didn't know for sure at the time, I was pretty convinced that I couldn't be the only one with this massive problem of forgetting whether I took my insulin.

With that idea in mind, I started reaching out to my peers, caregivers, and anybody associated in any way with diabetes to ask if this was a problem. The answer, overwhelmingly, was yes. Most people have forgotten their insulin injections often enough to create a big problem for them, and there was no good system for how to manage this. We heard about people trying to keep a daily diary, trying to position their insulin pens in a certain way in the refrigerator to help them remember, sticking the needle through a piece of paper on a calendar (not recommended), and a host of other ideas. The main theme was that there was no system that "worked." People with diabetes wanted a solution that didn't require learning any new complicated system, that wasn't bulky, that had no buttons to push, and that worked all the time. Developing this dream sounds like an easy task, but sometimes getting things to be incredibly simple can be incredibly difficult.

Leonardo da Vinci said, "Simplicity is the ultimate sophistication," and this was something that I was striving for. My middle brother, Andreas, and I started looking at different ideas for creating this simplicity in a product that would be affordable, would enhance life balance for those of us with diabetes, and most importantly, would be very easy to use. With his background in computer engineering, and as one of the co-creators of Skype, Andreas had experience using a concept called "heuristic design." It specifically involved examining the potential interface of the product/idea and judging its compliance with recognized usability principles (the "heuristics"). These principles, while seemingly obvious when you read them, are not necessarily obvious for many product designers. How often does it happen that you get a product that annoys you because it doesn't work perfectly? That is precisely what we were trying to avoid. We wanted to make sure that it used a menu system that was easily understood, that it gave immediate feedback that it was working, and that any unnecessary complication was stripped away.

Although the original concept for this idea came in June 2008, it wasn't until September 2010 that we formally started the company and kicked off the business idea behind it. Together with a third person, we founded ReCapsulin LTD, but we were forced to change the name because of a potential trademark infringement with a company producing an oral insulin treatment called "Capsulin." I was fortunate that my previous employer, Acceleration, was willing to let me scale down my time with them while starting to build "Timesulin." Acceleration agreed that I would work half-time for them and half-time on my own project. In reality, it's hard for me to work half-time on anything, so I would say more accurately that I had two full-time jobs at that stressful time in my life. By the way, I thought it would get easier once I was working only on Timesulin, but that was not the case. Launching a new business is hard work!

Timesulin is a replacement cap for your insulin pen that shows when you took your last insulin shot. When using this product, you will never miss an injection or accidentally double dose again. During that period, the team, with me in the CEO position, started building the business case around the idea and product. How long would it take to produce the product, which versions of insulin pens did we want to produce it for, what would it cost to produce it, and what was the regulatory framework for this potential medical device? The project required a lot of work to get it off the ground. Although incredibly busy and challenging, it was an extremely satisfying period in my life. As I started to become connected with the diabetes community, I was impressed with the dedication of those working at the diabetes charities, the global organizations like the International Diabetes Federation (IDF), people starting their own outreach programs, and the people I met daily who were just doing their very best to take care of their diabetes. The people I met were passionate about campaigning to raise awareness for diabetes and to make this chronic condition that we deal with every day a little easier to manage. Whether it was at the global, regional, national, or local levels, I was struck by the passion these people had to make the world better. What was inspiring for me, as a businessman entering this world of entrepreneurship, was how willing they were to help me and my business.

Of special note were two amazing people whom I came across, John Grummit, who is very active within Diabetes UK and, more recently, with the IDF where he sits on the board, and Paul Madden. (Incredibly, after being forwarded an email about the concept for Timesulin that I had sent to John Grummit, Paul remembered me from my days at Camp Joslin nearly fifteen years earlier.) These two people catapulted me into the diabetes community by introducing me to key influencers who could better help me understand if the problem of missed/double injections was truly serious. (Yes it is, as we know now.) They also helped to identify obstacles that we might encounter as we tried to build a company in this field, and features that were most desired by people living with diabetes every day. Perhaps, most importantly, they validated that we were working on something important. I recall some incredibly powerful words that Paul Madden sent to me when he first became aware of the project we were undertaking. His words played a key role in our decision to move ahead with the idea of Timesulin. Paul wrote this to me on March 24, 2011:

> I am happy to say that the few hundred thousand people I have worked with that have type 1 diabetes typically do not have diabetes on their mind as the most important thing. They have other wonderful life issues that they focus more energy on, while, at the same time, balancing their life with diabetes exceptionally well. Your concept is clearly a winner and I hope that I will have a chance to sit with you and learn a little more about this effort.

It was incredible to me, as a first-time entrepreneur with no experience in this entirely new field, who was bringing a new invention to market—especially a medical device!—to receive such encouragement from those around me. That email from Paul Madden provided the final incentive that motivated me to give up my "day job" and move ahead with this project. I thank him, and all the others, who supported us in the early days.

In terms of the success of launching Timesulin, I learned the importance of networking and very importantly, of listening closely to the advice of others who have experience. It may not always be that other people around you are right, but they will often approach a problem from a new perspective that you may not have thought about. To this day, I try to make time with at least one new person, every other week, who might be able to help. (Although, from the beginning, they might not necessarily appear able to add value.) By being open to new ideas and listening, we can learn a lot; we need to put ourselves into situations where we have a chance of being positively influenced.

Back to the story of Timesulin: Having received confirmation that an unmet need existed for those of us using insulin pens daily, our next step was to present the idea of Timesulin to a small group of investors who we thought would be willing to help fund the business. We looked for investors who would add valuable experience to the team, which at that early stage lacked any direct experience within the medical device field. One potential investor, in the early days, was a business acquaintance of my brother who had indicated an interest in our business. As part of her investigation into the company and our idea, this woman brought in an expert from within her own contact network who offered extensive experience working with medical devices to analyze the investment opportunity that Timesulin offered. We weren't prepared for all the detailed questions that our potential investor's advisor asked us, such as the commercialization strategy, regulatory environment, feasibility testing, patient surveys, and many questions that we hadn't even thought of yet. The amazing result: this powerhouse within the Swedish business landscape, an internationally recognized expert in the medical field, not only decided to participate in the investment round herself and bring along many people from her own network, but she even was willing to join the board of the company as Chair. We couldn't believe our luck in getting such a dynamic force to complement the team. It is with great satisfaction that we successfully raised the money that we needed to fund development of the product and allow Timesulin to enter the next stage of development...making a real product.

I left the security of my former company, a stable income, and what had been a successful career in digital marketing to follow my passion and risk everything to do something new. I felt so strongly that we had a winning idea that I was able to take a huge professional and personal risk to get this business off the ground, and I haven't regretted it to this day. That doesn't mean that it has been easy; it definitely hasn't. However, the satisfaction that I get from combining the excitement of building a new and vibrant company with our ability to truly help people live safer and more balanced lives with diabetes, is hugely satisfying and keeps me going every day.

With the company officially formed in September 2010, and the team "really" starting to work on the product in May 2011, it took us eight months to get our first version of a commercially ready product out the door. Using rapid prototyping techniques, we looked at all stages of the product lifecycle to try to reduce time to market as much as possible. Did we hit every aspect of our business plan that we said we would? Not necessarily, but we got close enough. I once heard that only 10% of new businesses started each year make it past year two. It's too early for us to know whether we will make it for sure, since we haven't passed that milestone yet, but all signs are pointing in the right direction. The wonderful customers whom we have so far are incredibly supportive. The feedback we've gotten from people of all ages tells us what a difference Timesulin has made in their diabetes management. It makes me tremendously proud. I admit that Timesulin doesn't solve all issues related to diabetes—far from it. However, our goal is to make one aspect of this thing that we live with every day just a little bit easier through smart innovation focused on super simple solutions. (For further information about Timesulin, please see the website at the conclusion of this chapter.)

So what does the future look like? As somebody who has lived with a chronic condition for most of my life, I have never been one to let it slow me down. On the contrary, I think that it has enhanced my determination to take responsibility and to be proud of what I do. Having been connected to this world of diabetes, and having spoken with thousands of people just like me, who live with diabetes every day, I am exploding with different ideas for making life just a little bit easier. I keep asking myself this question: If Apple can bring amazing new products like the iPad to the market, or if we can have cell phones that fit onto a watch, why don't we encounter more innovation for people living with diabetes or other chronic conditions? Let's work together to support small companies and people who really want to make a difference in this world of diabetes. By sharing experiences, learning from each other, and building strong and long-term relationships, we can do amazing things together. I love connecting with other people with diabetes. Find me on Twitter @johnsjolund. If you aren't already, I challenge you to get involved. If you are already involved, I challenge you to kick it up and do something new or different.

And *Vasaloppet*? I managed to dust myself off after my fall, survived a *hypoglycemic reaction* around four kilometers from the end, and finished the world's longest ski race. I wasn't first. But I also wasn't last! And the amount of pride that I felt receiving that medal was multi-dimensional. Don't let diabetes keep you from doing what you dream of. In fact, never let anything keep you from achieving your dreams. And if you plan to be in the north of Sweden on the first Sunday of March next year, please cheer for me as I again cross the *Vasaloppet* finish line.

www.timesulin.com

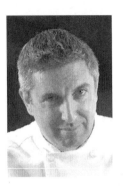

Photo credit by Charlie Brown

CHAPTER 23   *by Chris Smith, C.E.C.*

Recipe for Success

In 1993, I was attending the prestigious Culinary Institute of America (CIA), studying the skills needed to become a professional chef. My life was coming together, both professionally and personally. I began the year working, as part of my externship, at Le Cirque in New York City (one of the best fine-dining French restaurants in New York City) and was also newly engaged to my girlfriend. Until that time, I had been very healthy, with only a case of mononucleosis back in high school; more recently (January 1993), I was being treated for blood poisoning derived from what the doctor said was a spider bite. By February, I began to experience mild changes that would later be defined as symptoms. But I was not concerned about those subtle symptoms, considering my demanding lifestyle at the time. It was not until I lost a significant amount of weight in a very short time and went to the doctor again; I believed my life was in critical danger. I never would have guessed that with a new diagnosis, my life would continue and yet begin with a new sense of purpose. Looking back, I saw how close I had been to death and how my diagnosis was truly a blessing in disguise. This blessing would impact my cooking career in many ways and would allow me to serve others well beyond the kitchen walls that I envisioned. Ultimately, my life and career would take on a new level of meaning and focus to help others combat the epidemic of diabetes and obesity.

Experiencing what later was defined as a symptom, I began to feel fatigued throughout the day; I was always tired, which was quite the opposite of how I usually felt. However, I had a very demanding schedule that could explain why I was so tired.

Then there was the thirst. I was drinking from three to four gallons of liquids a day. From water to coffee and a variety of other liquids, I was trying to quench this never-quenchable thirst. I remember that, for a while, I was purchasing one-gallon jugs of juice (high sugar) because they were cheap; I was on a tight budget, and the juice had more flavor than water. I suspected that consuming that much liquid would result in my going to the bathroom often, and it did. I went back to the doctor when I began waking up every hour throughout the night. Soon after, I started having stomach cramps that were so severe that I again went back to the doctor's office, only to be misdiagnosed with an ulcer.

Those symptoms continued for about nine months, until I began to lose a significant amount of weight. I lost thirty pounds in six weeks, tipping the scale at 105 pounds. I walked into my doctor's office again, knowing that I was not well. I was twenty-seven years old, and I thought I was slowly dying. In fact, my mother (a registered nurse) shared with me years later that she had been concerned that I had stomach cancer. My only desire, when I walked into that doctor's office, was to know what was wrong and what I needed to do to feel normal again.

That time, my doctor simply pricked my finger and soon enough, he diagnosed me with diabetes. Because of my age, he was not sure if I had type 1 or type 2. I had little knowledge of diabetes. I had a childhood friend who had been diagnosed at a young age, and I recalled that he had had to urinate into a test tube and add a tablet that turned his urine a certain color. I also remember that he took shots, but that's as far as my knowledge went regarding diabetes.

As I asked questions, the doctor answered. I asked how diabetes would impact my culinary career. He was clear on the long-term effects of being on my feet for extended periods and of the stresses of being in a kitchen; he then recommended that I leave my career. I was twenty-seven years old and had just been told that, in order to live a life with few complications, I needed to leave the very career that I had prepared for my whole adult life. He arranged for me to be seen immediately for more blood work in the hopes of a more thorough checkup and a conclusive diagnosis. His words resonated with me as I drove to the hospital for more testing and for an accurate diagnosis. Although I was accustomed to thinking forward in my career and in life, I realized that I had to slow down. For now, I needed to be in the moment and to address what was going on right then: regaining my health.

After the doctor explained that I had diabetes, I asked what kind of diabetes I had. He explained that there are two types: type 1 (Juvenile Diabetes), which is usually diagnosed at a young age, and type 2 (Adult Onset), which is usually diagnosed later in life. He continued to say, "Type 1 can be managed with insulin shots, and type 2 can be managed with pills." Figuring that I didn't care for needles, and that I *was* older in diagnosis, I reassured my doctor that I probably had type 2 and that the pills would be fine! He just smiled and made an appointment for me to get further tests. I felt happy and relieved because I had convinced myself all the way to the hospital that I wouldn't need shots!

I arrived at the hospital, was seen, had blood worked up, and was officially diagnosed with type 1 diabetes (the one that I had to take shots for). I was sent to the seventh floor, where I was told to meet with someone who would educate me on what I needed to do next. I walked into the office of a Certified Diabetes Educator (CDE) whose office had a view of the Robert Moses Causeway, and I felt reassured that some things in life were about to change and others would remain the same. Like the bridge stretching over an impasse that leads to a new path, I too was coming to a bridge in my life. As the CDE helped me to understand diabetes, and how it would impact my life, she said something that would forever stay with me: "Diabetes is one of the few diseases you can control."

That statement was so powerful to me! I have control?? I have the ability to manage my disease and ultimately reduce the amount of complications that can occur with poor management? I can control my diabetes and not have diabetes control me! That was all I needed to hear.

My career? Not a problem, just manage your diabetes.

What about running or biking? Not a problem.

What about food - what can I eat? Not a problem, but I needed to be aware of how my body processed food and how it would relate to my diabetes management. I walked into that office unsure of where my bridge would lead me, but I walked out of that office determined not only to manage my diabetes but to continue my pursuit of becoming a professional chef.

Not knowing a lot about diabetes, I was eager to learn more, and I did. In time, I learned how to balance my diabetes (taking insulin, eating right, exercising, etc.) along with my personal and professional lives. I can honestly say that I have never had a day where I was angry or frustrated because of my diagnosis. Considering the alternative prior to diagnosis, I look at every day as a blessing and an opportunity. It's a blessing because I was diagnosed. The alternative, continuing to live without a diagnosis, clearly would have put my life and the lives of others around me in danger. (Currently one-third of all people affected with diabetes are not diagnosed. As of 2012, that equals eight million people in the United States alone.) The opportunity that resulted in my diagnosis was actually a message that we *all* can benefit from: be proactive and incorporate a healthy lifestyle by eating properly, exercising, managing stress, and continuing to work together with your healthcare team to best manage your personal health!

Recipe for Success: Person with Diabetes + Knowledge =
Better Management of Diabetes

That's how my life with diabetes began. My weight returned, although it took a few months; my thirst diminished to normal liquid consumption, and the cramps disappeared. I returned to the CIA and graduated that September as a C.E.C. (Certified Executive Chef). I was well educated on how to manage my diabetes, saw my endocrinologist on a quarterly basis, and began working as a chef in the hotel industry.

On one of my visits to my endocrinologist, he recommended that I teach a cooking class and demonstrate a simple recipe or two for their diabetes group. The group met every other month, and it sounded like a lot of fun; I agreed to demonstrate. I arrived early to organize and set up the room for a cooking demonstration. Because it was a clinical office, I had to set up my equipment, including the demonstration table, cook top, ingredients, recipes to distribute, etc. As people arrived, the forty chairs filled quickly, and there was standing room only. Just before I was introduced, I looked out to the audience and noticed that the back door was wide open. There were three heads, one on top of another, "looking in" because there was no additional room available. This really struck me, because I had not expected such a turnout, and neither had the endocrinology office! It was the largest attendance since the group had begun meeting!

The cooking demonstration went better than I could have imagined. Everyone was attentive and asked a lot of questions; yet as I spoke, there was a degree of seriousness in the audience that I was not expecting. Everyone was taking notes throughout the demonstration. I asked the audience how they would best describe the diabetic foods they currently ate and prepared. Their responses included *dry, tasteless, no flavor, and no variety*, just to name a few. They had more questions about portion size, carbohydrates, and salt intake. Honestly, it was a bit overwhelming. I was comfortable discussing food and all of its components that can support a healthy lifestyle, but I was surprised by the group's interest not only in food, but in their overall lifestyle and in how *all* things affected their blood glucose levels.

The evening was magical to me. As I drove home, my mind was racing with excitement. One aspect was reviewing the demonstration and then identifying areas that could help meet the needs that the audience had questions about! I realized that I could take my personal experience of having diabetes and merge it with my professional experience of being a chef. By the time I arrived home, I saw my life's mission in serving others. My plan was to be true to being a chef: use my creative outlet to develop healthier recipes that actually taste good and provide easy recipes that anyone can duplicate at home. I envisioned myself not only serving as a chef providing sustenance to the body, but also offering nourishment that truly helped to better manage the body.

By this time, I had graduated from the CIA, was newly married, and was currently working full-time at a four-star hotel. Wanting to start a family and move off of Long Island, I accepted an Executive Chef position with Marriott, which at the time was involved in healthcare, so we moved to my new job in North Carolina. Working full-time, starting a family, and managing my diabetes was the daily juggle—and I was enjoying my life.

One of the things I received after my diagnosis was a magazine called *Diabetes Forecast* published by the American Diabetes Association. In the 1990s, it was one of the few magazines dedicated to informing readers about all aspects of diabetes. One of the subjects included recipes. Eventually, I decided to call the publishers to ask if they needed any recipes and to offer my services as a chef. That one call, just on a whim, changed the course of my life. Peter Banks, Editorial Director of *Diabetes Forecast*, listened as I shared my story with him, and within a week, he asked if I would mind if the magazine told my story. A few months later, I was on the cover of the November issue of *Diabetes Forecast* magazine titled: "Chris Smith, The Diabetic Chef." We also agreed to work together and, as a result, I became an associate editor of the magazine and agreed to write some cookbooks as well. *Cooking with The Diabetic Chef* and *The Diabetic Chef's Year Round Cookbook* are currently available. I am currently cooking and writing my third cookbook.

Once the article came out, I began to receive calls from across the country requesting that I speak to their diabetes group or diabetes event. Within a very short time, I was invited to speak at nationally-recognized medical facilities and to healthcare professionals. This interest in my work had a snowball effect, and I began to see the ingredients of my vision coming together on how and where I (The Diabetic Chef) could share my knowledge and provide a realistic approach to cooking in the home. While the requests poured in, I was still working full-time at the hospital, balancing my home life with a new home and two young sons, and still managing my diabetes. In time I saw that I would have to make a decision to either stay in the corporate world or choose a riskier path and follow my passion as The Diabetic Chef. The answer to that question came to me one night as I spoke to an audience in Kansas City.

I was feeling really good that night. I had found my passion in sharing my story and demonstrating simple and easy ways to prepare healthy meals that most anyone can do. I enjoyed being in front of the audience and would often be close to the audience whether passing food in some stage of preparation or answering questions. I am up front and present. For me, standing behind a table and just cooking is not personal enough. Diabetes is very, very personal. It impacts not only the individual but the whole family in many ways, both obvious and not so obvious. I wanted to *speak to* my audience about my story and experiences, not *speak at* them. I wanted them to see me, to look into my eyes, and to know that I understood because I too am living with diabetes.

At the end of each program, I stayed and answered any additional questions they had; some simply thanked me for stopping by. As the crowd slowly dispersed and the last person came up to me, she said in a soft tone,

"Thank you, Chef Chris; you saved my son's life tonight." I smiled and graciously thanked her for her kind words, feeling slightly awkward and unsure about how to respond to such a profound statement. As she shook my hand in thanks, she said, "I am not sure you understand," and she turned around with my hand in hers and pointed to a frail looking man sitting in a seat a few rows back. "You see, my son was diagnosed at a very young age and, after many years of not being in control, he was developing complications. With feelings of frustration and hopelessness, he had given up on wanting to manage his diabetes. It was even a chore to convince him to come with me tonight. But he listened to you speak tonight, Chef Chris, and to how you shared your story and how you chose to live your life with diabetes. And, in you, he found the strength he needs to manage his diabetes again. So thank you, Chef Chris, and God bless." And, with that, she released my hand and left the program with her son.

I was amazed and awestruck at the same time. How could I have left such an impression? I had told my story many times, funny stories, quirky life stories. My cooking demonstration, although good, did not usually inspire that kind of a response. I caught up with the mom and son, spent some time with them, and wished him well on his renewed commitment to himself. When I arrived home from the event the next day, I had received an e-mail from the same woman, restating how thankful she was and how her son had turned a new leaf and was managing his diabetes and his life. I read the email one more time and decided to forward it to my parents with a note letting them know that I was making a difference by helping to make some lives a little bit better.

I eventually cut back on my role as Executive Chef in the healthcare field and focused my energies full-time in my role as The Diabetic Chef. I continued to travel throughout the U.S., demonstrating to the general public and healthcare professionals realistic ways to prepare healthy and nutritious food. I have more recently provided corporate wellness programs to many Fortune 500 companies, including Boeing, Coke®, Volvo, UPS®, Tyson® and Disney®. In addition, 2013 will start off with a new cooking venue on the high seas on Holland America®, where I will continue to teach healthy cooking as we sail to the South African coast and Brazil.

Since I began my work as The Diabetic Chef, one thing is clear: the work became my life's mission, and that mission is so much bigger than I had ever envisioned. (For more information on The Diabetic Chef, please see the website at the end of this chapter.) I had hoped to inspire an interest in healthy cooking, never thinking that I would be seen as a source of inspiration for other people living with diabetes. I never expected this job to take on that kind of role. Yet my experiences over the years have confirmed my belief that I am doing the work I was meant to do, and I am proud to be someone who can help make a difference in other people's lives. It is my wish, when I look back many years from now, to know that I have helped many, have provided the spark of inspiration to overcome any limitations, and have offered a little hope to those who might have lost sight of how special we all are. Some might see that as a blessing in disguise; I believe that it's a blessing in plain sight.

www.TheDiabeticChef.com

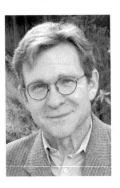

CHAPTER 24   *by Jim Turner*

The Gift

On February 9, 1970, I was diagnosed with what we called Juvenile Diabetes in the old days. I was a junior at Herbert Hoover High School in Des Moines, Iowa. I was seventeen years old.

I don't know if you remember being seventeen. I do. It arrived as I staggered away from my totally clueless, anxious, nerve-wracking sixteenth year. And for me, sixteen was very blue. I was hoping, *praying*, that when I turned seventeen, things would suddenly somehow get a lot better. Boy, did they ever not. I remained a clunky, uncomfortable, awkward, clodhopping, unsure-of-himself stick of dynamite.

The spice I added to that rancid soup when I got to seventeen was a painful, hyper-self-awareness of all the changes that were cluttering up my body—but, of course, without the benefit of my understanding any of them. While hormones ravaged my body, acne attacked my face. Every day as I walked to school, I was positive that the Soviets were going to drop a nuclear bomb on me. Just on me. They didn't. Somehow, I outlasted the Soviet Empire.

I really was a total mess. But most of us were. Even though a handful of my classmates seemed comfortable in the skin they found themselves in, I can assure you (having just attended my fortieth high school reunion) that many just hid their fears and frustrations better than the rest of us. Months after turning seventeen, on top of everything else that was happening with my revolting body (by that, I mean revolting *against* me), it now started to fall apart. And I mean literally fall apart.

Not only was the typical teenage war going on inside me, against me, but now my "me" started to wither and die. I lost thirty pounds off an already skinny frame. I was ravenous all the time. Every day at school, I would eat two lunches and top if off with three or four giant peanut butter cookies—none of which satisfied my hunger. I basically had one meal: It started in the morning with two giant bowls of cereal and didn't end until I fell asleep. I ate all day long and felt as though I was starving to death (which I actually was).

I had no energy. Acne starting growing on top of my acne. My thirst was unquenchable. I drank water until my stomach felt like bursting.

And…I'd urinate.

Oh my, the urination. I urinated and urinated and urinated, until it seemed I couldn't possibly urinate another drop, but I could. And did. And did. And did. The urinating was finally the key to discovering what was wrong with me.

I didn't actually see my parents that much in those days. Seventeen-year-olds do not like hanging out with mom and dad, but I was also doing whatever I could to hide my condition. I was wretchedly embarrassed about every single thing about me, every minute, of every day.

My folks and I all left the house at different times. When I was at home, I mostly hung out in my basement bedroom—with a ping-pong table and fireplace and stereo—listening to music and drinking gallons of water. At night, I'd go out with friends to Dairy Queen, McDonalds®, places like that. But one night, I came out of my cave to have dinner with my parents and younger brother and sister. As we sat there at the dinner table, my dad said to me—and he was really embarrassed to say this—he said, "Jim, uh… when you get up to urinate in the middle of the night, try to have a little, um, better aim. You're kind of spraying everywhere."

I said, "I'm getting up like ten times a night to urinate."

There was a pause in the discussion. Actually, the discussion screeched to a halt. Now… we lived in a two-story house. Everyone else's bedrooms were on the top floor. My bedroom was in the basement. The bathroom I used was on the main floor, and ten times a night, I would trudge up the stairs to urinate.

That night, my mom lay awake in bed all night listening to me trudge up those stairs to go to the bathroom. The next morning, she called a kidney specialist, and I went in to see him that day. The kidney specialist took one look at me and told me that I probably had that Juvenile Diabetes thing. He set up an appointment for me to see a diabetes specialist the next day. That night, the whole family went out to dinner for my grandmother's sixtieth birthday.

I didn't know anything about diabetes except that I might have to maybe take shots. But the one thing I was absolutely positive about was that I would never be able to eat sugar again, ever. This I was sure of. So I treated this event as if it were my death-row meal. I ordered every dessert they had—since I would never, ever be able to eat sugar again or have another dessert FOR THE REST OF MY LIFE. I was going to leave dessert behind in a blaze of glory.

The other thing that squirmed in a little corner in the back of my mind was this thing about shots: a concept about which I had to do all sorts of mental gymnastics to keep very far from my thoughts.

The next day, I went to see a stern but warm doctor (with a wonderfully quirky sense of humor) who did some tests and then told me that, yes, I did have Juvenile Diabetes. It turned out that my blood sugar was *over* 1000 mg/dL! *"Why was I not in a coma?"* He sent me home to get some clothes for a week in the hospital and told me that he was going to train me how to "be a diabetic." *"What? TRAIN me to 'be a diabetic'?"* As I drove away, my main thought was that I wasn't crazy. Something was wrong with me. It had a name. At that point, I didn't even think about the treatment. I'd forgotten about the shots. I was just happy to know that the horrible feeling had a name.

So I went home and got some clothes, my homework, and some books. My folks dropped me off at the hospital. They didn't have any rooms available, so I got placed in a big pediatric/orthopedic ward with lots of kids in traction. It was very weird—all those kids with broken legs, necks, backs—everyone hanging in straps and pulleys…and then me. A nurse came over carrying a tray with a tiny bottle of medicine and a syringe. She drew up a dose of the medicine, gave me a shot, and said, "This is what you'll be taking from now on." All the kids starting groaning and yelling, "Oh nooo, shots! Look at that poor sucker!"

I sat in my bed for a long time, feeling sorry for myself. All those kids were going to get out of their traction, but I was going to have to take shots forever. *"F-O-R-E-V-E-R."* The thought of that was overwhelming. Plus I still felt sick, as though I had some kind of rotten energy-draining flu.

Nothing about it seemed fair. I was miserable. But then, after about an hour, a funny thing happened: I started to feel good. I started to feel like what I remembered feeling human felt like. I probably hadn't felt good for months, even though it seemed like years. And now I could feel myself emerging from a daze. I felt good. And boy, did it feel good to feel good.

I went over to the nurse who gave me the shot and said, "Whatever it was that you just gave me… I want that."

She said, "That was just insulin."

And I said, "Well, that's what I want."

That first shot of insulin was a dramatic introduction to the first of many tools that I would collect over the years to co-exist with the "800-pound gorilla" that followed me everywhere. As I said to the nurse, "That's what I want." That tiny bottle was salvation to me. I didn't even mind the delivery system.

Of course, I would later have relationship issues with this glorious drug. Hello, *hypoglycemia*! But from the beginning, I was happy to take the shots. The wretched feeling of high blood sugar was all the motivation I needed. Looking back, I see how lucky I was to be driven to learn how to control the "diabetes ape." To this day, I still hate the feeling of high blood sugar, and I'm quick to correct it (sometimes too quick to correct it, and my blood sugar ends up yo-yoing).

The first thing I wanted to do was learn how to use this wonderful tool. It frustrated me that the nurses knew how to do this and I didn't. So I learned how to give myself shots as soon as I could. Another tool. And that's not saying that it wasn't scary at first. I suffered through my share of failures. A nervous tic that I had at first made me plunge the syringe into my leg and then pull it out before I could give the dose. I wrote this off as ramped-up, nervous energy.

When I finally perfected the shot-giving, I felt…large. Besides finally feeling good, I felt in control of my body—something I hadn't felt in a long, long time and a feeling that is alien to most seventeen-year-olds, whether they have diabetes or not.

My memories of that week in the hospital learning how to "be a diabetic" are good ones. I was excited to learn from my mistakes while gaining some measure of self-respect by actually gaining control over an aspect of my adolescent body.

Luck played a part in all this too. I was very lucky that I didn't end up in a coma with my blood sugar over 1000 mg/dL. Secondly, I was just miraculously lucky to be introduced to diabetes by the doctor who diagnosed me: Dr. Edward Hertko, my first diabetes hero—who completely understood the rough and tumble nature of this disease—a man who understood that the sooner the patient got the keys to the car, the better, so to speak.

The day I checked out of the hospital, Dr. Hertko dropped a bomb on my mom and me. As my dad signed the discharge papers, my mother said to Dr. Hertko, "What can I do for Jimmy?" Dr. Hertko stood up. He was six-foot four-inches tall and exuded a do-not-screw-with-me vibe like no one I've ever met. He said, "What can YOU do for Jimmy? You can put three meals a day on the table and *stay out of the way*. If Jim doesn't figure this disease out, we've all got trouble."

And he was out the door and on his way to saving another family years of anguish.

My mother is still alive, and so is Dr. Hertko—both in their eighties—and to this day, she's still a little skittish whenever she asks me a question about my diabetes. She looks around as though Dr. Hertko might come crashing out of the ceiling.

This was the gift that I received. By throwing the whole kit and kaboodle in my lap, Dr. Hertko gave me the best gift any person with diabetes can receive: hands-on control of my disease. MY disease. He showed me that I would control it only if I owned it. He put the responsibility on me. Dr. Hertko said he would be there to give directions, show me the tools, and point the way—but it was up to me to do the heavy lifting. At times, it has been very heavy lifting, but nothing has had more to do with my excellent control of my diabetes. Nothing.

I've heard too many nightmare stories about doctors who told their patients that they needed to cut back on their lives because they have diabetes. Dr. Hertko never once told me that I couldn't do something. He told me that I could do everything.

After high school, I headed out into the world. I loved travel and was happy to do oddball job after oddball job (cabbie, school janitor, ice cream scooper, roofer, doll eye maker, etc.) to make enough money for another journey.

On one of my many bicycle trips, a friend and I rode for three months around England, Scotland, Belgium, Germany, Holland, Austria, Switzerland, and Italy. In Switzerland, my friend got hit by a car and flew home a week later. I continued alone, riding the length of Italy by myself to visit relatives in Calabria. That was in 1973, and home blood sugar testing was still a faraway dream—a tool a decade away. I rode thousands of miles all over Europe for three months and never once knew the level of my blood sugar.

I eventually stumbled (literally) into the theater department at the University of Iowa and wound up in a comedy group that still survives almost forty years later. This led to a long and continuing career in acting and comedy.

Since first jumping onto the show business bandwagon in 1975, I've done dozens of movies (from *The Right Stuff* to *Bewitched*); I've been a regular on several television series, most notably seven years on HBO's *ARLI$$*; I ran for president in 1988 on MTV as a hippy character whom I created: "Randee of the Redwoods." This past year, I've guest-starred on *Boston Legal, Big Bang Theory, Franklin & Bash, Happy Endings, Castle, Undercovers, Young & The Restless, Party Down*—all while carrying my tool box of tools that I carry proudly every single day, every hour, every minute of my life. That and the gift of responsibility that Dr. Hertko laid at my doorstep four decades ago.

I turned sixty this year. I play basketball several times a week, walk, play golf, lift weights, and am in better shape than most of my peers. One of the younger guys (actually they're all younger; I'm the oldest by years) in one of my basketball games recently said to me, "You're so lucky to have diabetes. You have to take such great care of your body. Kudos to your health."

Years ago, I heard through the grapevine that some people were going to do a show about people living with diabetes, and it was going to be done by people living with diabetes. The name of the show in development was "*dLife*." I tracked down the producers and told them, "You will not find a better person for this job."

And even though it never got to that point, I would've arm-wrestled anybody for that job. Fortunately, I never had to; eight years later, and I'm still there. It's like I've come full circle.

As my friend said, "You're lucky to have diabetes."

I couldn't agree more. It's the gift that keeps on giving.

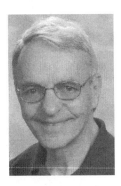

CHAPTER 25   *by Saul Zuckman*

Welcome to the Team

I have been a person with type 2 diabetes since 1990. I had just started a new job very shortly before I was diagnosed, and neither my employer nor the insurance company was thrilled by the event. I was too new with the company for my feelings to be considered. However, I was now at the crossroads, and it was time to reach deep to see "what I was made of." I was successful in negotiating through the required compliance steps to take control. This included losing seventy-nine pounds over three years and adjusting my attitude and expectations regarding the disease. My greatest internal challenge was asking for and accepting assistance and help from those near and dear to me. This included anyone who was making the effort to control their diabetes. I learned from both those who were successful and from the experiences of those who were struggling to gain control. I quickly learned that, although diabetes is a chronic disease with no cure currently available, it is well understood by the medical and scientific community. The medications and technology are continually improving. Our control can be improved by adhering to the advice we receive: take medication/insulin as directed, lose weight (if required), exercise on a regular basis, eat more fruits and vegetables, and watch those calories and carbohydrates as well as portion sizes.

On this journey, I met several incredible people. I was inspired by those with greater challenges, and I had the opportunity to help empower others to do "the right things." Although it was frustrating at times, "it was all good." What do I think about having diabetes? Well, if I had my choice, I would rather not have this or any other chronic disease. However, if I were forced to choose a chronic disease, I would choose diabetes. As I see it, diabetes does respond to control principles and practices (compliance, compliance, compliance), and we have the opportunity to take charge and to improve ourselves and those who surround us. Diabetes allowed me to meet a circus clown up close and personal, to interact with incredible people, and to get an upgraded racing bicycle.

My Diagnosis

Certainly, we all remember the circumstances and events that led to being diagnosed with diabetes. My experience, however, was really embarrassing. Although I was very overweight, or maybe obese, I did not experience the classic symptoms of unexplained weight loss, an unquenchable thirst, fatigue, and the constant urge "to go" that drives many to their healthcare professionals for medical attention. Then, how did I get there?

On a November afternoon in 1990, I went with a few co-workers to the mall food court for lunch. It was National Diabetes Awareness Month, and one of the major medical teaching universities in my area was offering free diabetes screenings and blood pressure testing. They had correctly anticipated that only a few people would volunteer for the test and screening. So, to encourage greater participation, they hired circus-type clowns to mingle with the lunchtime crowd to encourage people to come to the testing stations.

Four of us were seated at my table, and one clown came over, zeroed in on me, and ignored the others; the others were annoyed and amused. They encouraged me to go and get tested, figuring that it might be a good idea *and* that we would get rid of the clown and his annoying antics. The clown won, and I followed him to the testing station to get my blood pressure taken and to leave a sample of blood to be tested for diabetes. I completed a short medical questionnaire and was told that the results would be sent to my healthcare professional within ten days.

I received a call from my doctor two weeks later, suggesting that I come in to see him. I asked the doctor why he was calling and if there was a problem with the clown's diabetes test. He said he was not sure but thought it would be a good idea if I came to his office to discuss the data and to take some additional tests.

With a great deal of apprehension, I went into my doctor's office first thing Monday morning. After a brief interview and a finger stick test, along with the "clown report," he said he had no doubt that I had type 2 diabetes. However, he wanted a professional laboratory test to confirm the findings, and boy did it ever! The lab result showed my blood sugar was *over* 400 mg/dL after a nine-hour fast. Plus, my hemoglobin A1c, which shows the blood glucose average over the previous two to three months, was also high—in fact, it was in excess of 12%, which is nearly double the normal range.

The A1c test is extremely important, especially if the results indicate high blood sugar levels over an extended period of time. High blood sugars may increase the risk of developing diabetes complications such as blindness, leg amputations, heart disease, or even death. That's why the American Diabetes Association (ADA) urges us to strive to maintain an A1c level below 7%, and many healthcare professionals would like to see their patients strive for blood glucose levels of 6.5%. I guess the clown was right, and he may have done me a favor by embarrassing me into taking the screening.

Yup, I certainly had type 2 diabetes. I quickly understood that diabetes is a chronic, lifetime disease. Yet, while there may not be a cure at this time, the disease is well understood and can be controlled with medication (which may include insulin), exercise, healthy food choices, portion control, and weight management. The risks and rewards were my choice. Now it was time to create my success plan to manage my disease.

My first step was to tell my world that I was a person with diabetes, and I was not going to hide it or apologize for it. The next step was to understand what I was dealing with and to convince myself that, although diabetes is serious, it's not a death sentence. Education and the knowledge about my diabetes were certainly as powerful as the treatment plan. Approximately one in nine people in our country has diabetes, which is just about 11%. But, alarmingly, about a third more are just like I was; they have diabetes but are not yet diagnosed. An estimated fifty-four million people in this country have *pre-diabetes*. Maybe they need to see the clown!

Some of the best experts I found were those who were already experiencing the disease. I searched and found diabetes support groups whose members inspired me with their successes. What I learned was that diabetes care was in my control. Those who empowered themselves and embraced the principles of diabetes compliance, spelled out by healthcare professionals, were extremely successful in managing their diabetes.

These concepts were important, but I wasn't sure if I needed to start my diabetes care *immediately* on the heels of being diagnosed. I probably had had this disease for several prior years. It really didn't hurt, so why not wait a few months before getting started? I thought, *"I have enough to deal with today."*

My Promise

But the option to delay taking control was short circuited by my four-year-old grandson. We were playing with blocks when he unexpectedly looked me square in the face and asked, "Grandpa, are you going to die? I don't want you to die." Where did this come from? I was surprised that he knew what death was.

Then, I realized that my daughter and son-in-law must have been talking about it in their home. Sure, in their eyes I was getting on in years, significantly overweight, and now had diabetes. This was the trifecta for disaster.

After regaining my composure, I assured my grandson that I would be around for a long, long, time to come. I told him that I would watch him grow up and even have great grandchildren. I told him that I was going to look after my health, lose weight, exercise, and do all the necessary things to control my diabetes. That satisfied him, and he returned to his playing without further comments. With that, I stroked my chin and asked myself, *"How do I keep this promise?"* I needed to get my diabetes and health under control starting right then!

My treatment plan started with an introductory dose of oral hypoglycemic medication and a trip to the dietitian, who was retiring the next day. She all but emptied her subject-matter file drawer into my lap and wished me luck by saying, "I hope you find some of this helpful." She gave me a list of some very boring foods and a tutorial on food exchanges and the importance of portion control. I was convinced that she was trying to starve me. If that wasn't enough, she required moderate aerobic physical exercise for thirty minutes per day, most days of the week.

My doctor wanted me to check back with the diabetes educator in two weeks. On the next visit, I was seen by a Certified Diabetes Educator (CDE) new to the practice. She was a lot more supportive, and she celebrated my successes. She invited my wife to join in on the sessions; with new resolve, and my wife's commitment of support, we immediately started on a new regimen of healthy food and exercise.

I returned for the follow-up appointment, and to the diabetes educator's surprise, my glucose readings were in the normal range for people without diabetes. The doctor came in, reviewed that data, and then asked, "What have you done?" I told him that I had eaten only the boring foods on the list, almost starved myself with the meager portion allowance, bought a new pair of running shoes, and hit the road most days of the week. My legs were still rubbery.

I said to the doctor, "I guess that was a 'magic pill' you prescribed." He assured me that the purpose of the dose of oral medication was to see if I could tolerate the active ingredient and that it was not the reason that the blood sugar was under control. He took me off the medication and went with the lifestyle adjustments alone. He warned that diabetes was a progressive disease and that I might need to take oral medications—or even insulin—in the future, despite compliance to instructions that had been effective. For the time being, my mantra was "compliance, compliance, compliance."

This session led me to a visit with Tom, a pharmacist friend of mine, who owned and operated an independent drug store. I told him that I wanted to learn more about medications for diabetes. Tom briefed me on the available oral medications and how they worked. That conversation did not take all that long. The year was 1991, and we had only a few classes of oral medications compared to what is available today. Tom said that he had something else to show me, but warned that I might be offended. With that said, Tom took a small box from his refrigerator that contained a vial of insulin. I looked at it and said, "I hope that my diabetes never gets to be so bad that I would need insulin." I considered insulin to be the treatment of last choice and maybe the end of the road. Tom pointed out that insulin was an effective means of keeping blood sugar under control and that using it did not mean that my diabetes was getting worse.

Insulin is a hormone that is formed naturally by the body. Type 2 diabetes is caused by insufficient insulin production from beta cells, which results in insulin resistance. Type 2 diabetes is characterized by *progressive* beta-cell failure. Some people with type 2 diabetes require only oral medications for treatment. Other people will need to add insulin, or another injectable medication, because their blood sugar levels are not controlled. The addition of a *basal* insulin is not indicative of failure. The quality of today's laboratory-produced insulin is close to that made by nature. Tom pulled the product information sheet from a vial of insulin, and I noticed that insulin had been around for over seventy-five years, much longer than the oral medication had.

Things went well for the next five years, except for the weight gain. When I was diagnosed, I was a bit overweight. I think I may have let my guard down because my weight increased into the obese range as measured by the BMI. However, I still felt good, and nothing hurt. Despite my careful food choices (except for the size of the portions) and an aggressive exercise program, my fasting blood sugar continued to increase.

My doctor was concerned that if these high numbers continued to stay high over time, I would suffer from diabetes complications. He gave me a prescription for an oral medication and suggested that I visit a dietitian/diabetes educator. I thought about asking him about insulin, but at the last minute decided to give the oral medication a try. I rationalized that if I increased my exercise (although I had no idea how that would be possible), I would not have to see the dietitian/diabetes educator.

I stuck to my plan for several months. Things started to improve somewhat, but my blood glucose levels remained above the desired range. My A1c was just above 8%, well beyond my goal. On the next visit to my doctor, we agreed that this plan was not working and discussed trying a different medication. With my doctor's guidance, I tried several oral diabetes medications, but they weren't effective. I experienced several more months of marginal control, which I feared would increase the risk of complications. I did not want to continue that risk. I told my doctor about Tom and my promise that I would go on insulin once diet, exercise, and lifestyle changes were no longer effective. I then asked him what he thought about insulin at that time. He looked a little surprised and told me that we had not yet exhausted the pre-insulin options.

Time for Insulin

He assured me that insulin would work and asked whether I was sure that I wanted to use it. I assured him that this was an informed decision. Over time, I learned about the insulin pump, which is an alternative to daily injections and allows for intensive insulin therapy when used in conjunction with blood glucose monitoring and carbohydrate counting. I believed that this would make a significant contribution to my "taking control" strategy, considering my commitment to increase my exercise.

I took the idea of going on an insulin pump back to my healthcare team for their thoughts. My doctor said that he wasn't familiar with pump technology, and he thought it would be better to switch my diabetes care to an endocrinologist who was familiar with the pump; he then gave me a referral. Initially, I thought I would need to build a new healthcare team, but that was not the case. The endocrinology group limited their practice to matters of metabolism, which included diabetes, and my doctor handled the rest.

My team had now grown, and these professionals were a welcome addition to my team. My endocrinologist understood my desire to maintain tight control by going on the insulin pump, but he wanted to hold off until he saw how I reacted to standard therapy. Although he would not authorize the pump at that point, he did introduce me to the insulin pen which made things much more convenient.

Several months later, and after much nagging on my part, he did authorize the use of the pump, which was very expensive. My health insurance covered only a minimal amount, but I believed it was worth the investment. After the usual number of start-up issues, I was successful and did well using the pump. The most significant issue was pumping Regular insulin, since rapid acting insulin had not yet been introduced. The onset time for Regular insulin is thirty minutes, and it has a duration of six to eight hours. The pump injects *basal* insulin, small bursts of insulin between meals to mimic the healthy body dealing with sugar released from the liver. This makes calculating *bolus* dosages challenging because, if I miscalculated, then I might experience a low blood sugar reaction. Yet, through trial and error, I settled into a routine fairly quickly.

My experience with the pump helped keep my blood sugar levels under tight control. The pump—along with exercise, food choices, portion control, carbohydrate counting, frequent testing, and compliance, compliance, compliance—kept my A1c below 6% without significant *hypoglycemic* events.

However, the journey was not seamless. The pump does require operating overhead, such as addressing mechanical issues, changing infusion sets, filling the reservoir, and charging the battery. It is desirable to carry a pump spare-parts kit along with a backup syringe and vial of insulin when being away from the supply center for more than twenty-four hours. The results are certainly worth the effort.

A1c Champions

I registered on the Aventis Pharmaceutical website, which offered information on diabetes. Shortly after, I received a telephone call from Patient Mentor Institute (PMI), a peer-to-peer diabetes education organization. They were looking for volunteers to be "A1c Champions" for a non-product-specific taking-control program for people who had diabetes. Through this experience, I learned to respect my diabetes and to no longer fear it, since I was confident that I could take control.

Next, I had the opportunity to travel throughout the United States, making our carefully scripted presentations to encourage taking control of diabetes. Each audience gave us a special reception, realizing that we were in this together. Also, the cadre of A1c Champions bonded almost instantly into a loving, inspiring, and caring family.

During my presentations, I spoke of the support I received from my wife and the commitment to physical exercise—especially long-distance bicycle riding. I had progressed to the point where I was able to increase my exercise intensity to "moderate" at least ninety minutes per day, most days of the week. Riding my bicycle became very special to me, and it grew to the point where I owned six bicycles. I completed several aggressive multi-day rides, but nothing that could be considered competitive.

Race Across America

Then, at one of our PMI training update meetings, I learned that Sanofi-Aventis was forming a bicycle racing team where each of the riders had type 2 diabetes. The bicycle athletic team was under Team Type 1, Inc. of Atlanta, GA. Team Type 2 was to participate in Race Across America (RAAM), which is a 3,005-mile bicycle race from Oceanside, CA (near San Diego) to Annapolis, MD. This race was viewed as one of the toughest endurance events on the face of the earth since it was a non-stop event across the entire country.

I was asked if this would interest me, and the good news was that it would fulfill one of my "bucket list" items. Imagine seeing the country from the seat of a bicycle! The bad news was that I would need to resign from the A1c

Champions program because the corporate policy didn't allow me to participate in both programs. As much as I loved and enjoyed the A1c Champions program, I just could not set aside the bicycling Team Type 2 opportunity. I promptly filed my resignation and made application to Team Type 2.

The parent organization, Team Type 1, was founded by two young bicycling enthusiasts, Phil Sutherland and Joe Eldridge, both of whom were persons with type 1 diabetes. Phil had conceived the idea during his college years when he heard people telling him what he could not do because he had diabetes. Phil knew that he had to find a way to prove to the doubters (and to himself) that having diabetes does not make you a second-class citizen to be pitied or patronized. Phil believed that the best way to do this would be to form a team of athletes with diabetes and to enter and win RAAM.

Phil and Joe made this their highest priority. The first year's attempt, in 2006, drew a lot of attention from the bicycling community and healthcare professionals. The team raced across the country, 3,042.8 miles, in five days, sixteen hours, and four minutes—just three minutes behind the winning team. The finish line for the 2006 RAAM was the Atlantic City, NJ boardwalk. The goal was to show that people with diabetes who were properly trained and were carefully monitoring and controlling their blood sugar, could accomplish what others without diabetes could do.

Later, they formed another team to show that people with type 2 diabetes, who were typically older, could, with proper training and diabetes compliance, do what others without diabetes could do and maybe a little bit faster. The plan was to field a team of persons with type 2 diabetes to compete in the RAAM. Phil was realistic in his expectations and did not expect Team Type 2 to win their class (eight-person team) or to set new course records. Denny, one of our two road captains, challenged each member of the team to complete the race without wandering off, without getting lost, and without dying. He would consider this feat a success.

But Team Type 2 did much better than that. They competed in both the 2009 and 2010 RAAM in the category of eight-rider teams and finished faster than the last team to finish—but not by much. Setting all excuses aside, Team Type 2 was the oldest team in the race, competing against nine other eight-man teams, including Team Type 1 and the European teams with Olympic-quality athletes. I was the most senior aged rider on Team Type 2 and, in fact, at age seventy, the oldest finisher in all of RAAM in 2010. My age increased the average age of the team by about two years. In fact, we were old enough to be the parents of the Team Type 1 "kids."

Now for the question before Team Type 1 management: How does one get a team of senior citizens across the country safely? If successful, that would send a loud message that people with type 2 diabetes, given proper conditioning and full compliance, can exceed the abilities of people without diabetes. The game plan was team training and conditioning. However, if a team member became seriously ill or worse during the race, the entire message would be lost, and the team might dissolve in embarrassment.

The training would take about eight months, led by Tim Henry, a professional bicycle coach and racer from Atlanta. Although he himself was not a person with diabetes, he was fully conversant in the issues of athletes with diabetes. He had considerable experience with Team Type 1 athletes. However, they were elite athletes and much younger than those in his current challenge. Most of Team Type 2 had never participated in a competitive bicycle event. These athletes would need to go through a boot camp of training plus learn how their diabetes would react to the vigorous training and ultimately the competition.

Tim's plan included working with us on endurance, conditioning, and nutrition. The training regimen was customized for each of us and administered through a training website that Tim updated weekly. He was successful in getting the team at peak performance for the start of the race. The team also had monthly group telephone calls to exchange information and enhance team member bonding. Although some of us never really met each other until the start of the race in Oceanside, CA, we felt the "love" and were never strangers.

As we approached the RAAM start date, the training intensity was rolled back, but the duration increased. Sometimes the training was four hours per day and on consecutive days. When we started receiving the countdown instructions from team management and our coach, the excitement ramped up. We packed up to ride and received expressions of well wishes and encouragement from our teammates who were not racing this year and from folks who were following us on Facebook and the Team Type 1 website. (For further information about Team Type 1, please see the website at the conclusion of this chapter). My wife did not accompany me but stayed at home, cheered the team, and followed the progress on the team site. Our local media sought out many of us for feature and human-interest stories. My story was published in the local media and in the telephone directory. This was the real deal.

Three days before the start of the race, we flew to San Diego International Airport, then shuttled to the local Holiday Inn Express in Oceanside, CA. A week before, we had forwarded our bicycles to the hotel. The race coordination was huge and took on a military-style precision. Supporting a bicycle team to race across the country was a mammoth feat. When you added to the mix the challenge that each member of the team also needed to control his diabetes, it increased the challenge. Our racing team had eight riding members, plus a crew of twenty-one support people, two RVs, and four SUVs. The crew consisted of drivers, navigators, cook and kitchen staff, and even a licensed masseuse who gave each of us three deep-tissue massages per day. We also had constant access to a doctor specializing in athletes with diabetes. The entire crew was dedicated, encouraging, and very supportive.

The race was relay style and continued around the clock until we crossed the finish line in Annapolis, MD. As we raced, we crossed the Palomar Mountain and Laguna Coastal Ranges and started heading in a northeasterly direction in Arizona for a distance of 3,005 miles. This included the Rocky Mountains and many of the other challenging mountain ranges across the country. We split our eight-man team into two four-person squads that we named "Tango" and "Cash" after the movie of the same name with Sylvester Stallone and Kurt Russell. Each squad would ride eight-hour shifts, rotating one racer at a time to the road. The other squad would be riding in one of our two RVs, getting a hot meal, shower, massage, and maybe some sleep while being shuttled to the transition point where the on-the-road squad would be ending their shift.

We knew at the start of the race that there would be significant challenges to control our diabetes and to deal with sleep deprivation and the obvious factors of speed, strength, and stamina. The beginning of the race was fueled by excitement and the adrenalin rush. But it didn't take long to start seeing the effects of endurance exercise on our diabetes. I was the first on Squad Cash to be caught by low, really low, blood sugars. All during our squad's eight-hour shift, the two of us on insulin pumps reduced our meal time *bolus* and *basal* infusion to accommodate the vigorous level of activity. Our squad increased our caloric intake with protein and high glycemic food and hydrated almost continually with water, energy drinks, and electrolyte products. At the end of our shift, we turned the racing over to Squad Tango for the next eight hours.

I had lowered my *basal* and *bolus* doses during our shift and consumed what I thought to be "too many calories." My blood glucose numbers had somewhat increased during the shift, which I believed to be overcompensating for the activity. The dinner meal was going to be protein and high carbohydrate. I had increased my *basal/bolus* slightly, thinking that I would need the insulin to match the carbohydrate intake. However, about three hours after the meal, I felt the onset of a *hypoglycemic* event. I went for my meter to test, but before I could lance my finger, the blood sugar low had taken over, and I was quickly losing the ability to care for myself. I began to act irrationally.

My teammate, Tony, recognized what was happening and quickly took charge. He took a blood sugar reading, although I argued with him that I was "just fine" and did not need help. It was 27 mg/dL, and Tony immediately started to administer any type of simple carbohydrate he could get his hands on. There were plenty of glucose tablets and simple carbohydrates in the RV. His concern was that I would lose consciousness. We did not have *glucagon* in the van at that time, but we made sure to get it within the hour. My blood sugars quickly responded to the infusion of carbohydrates. We may have overcorrected because my blood sugar increased to over 200 mg/dL. Thanks to Tony's knowledge and quick reaction, a more serious event was averted. Tony, by the way, was a September 11th First Responder, and I could certainly see why.

The Finish Line

As the race progressed, it was apparent that our team would not make a significant impact on the race results. We were fighting to not finish in last position. However, during the course of the race, Team Type 2 did have opportunities to advance our mission of showing the benefits of taking control of your diabetes with age not being a limiting factor. We drew media attention across the nation and the admiration of many who came out to support us. We had the opportunity to chat with those who were new to diabetes, veterans of the disease, family and friends in support of a person(s) with diabetes, and those who were just curious.

A significant moment came at Penalty Box Time Station #52 in Mt. Airy, MD, which was fifty-five miles from the end of the race. Squad Tango was serving the fifteen-minute penalty, and Squad Cash had moved onto the finish line in Annapolis. The race would end outside of Annapolis, and all team members would then ride together to the ceremonial finish next to the Naval Academy. It was about 2 a.m. when we arrived at the Penalty Box Time Station. We were greeted by a mother and her nine-year-old son, Lester, who had been diagnosed with type 1 diabetes a few weeks earlier. Mom explained that Lester was having a difficult time accepting his diagnosis and that his classmates at school were teasing him about having to go to the school nurse for testing, administering insulin, and having to eat a snack mid-morning and mid-afternoon. This level of negative attention was starting to get Lester down and had him questioning his self-worth. She had brought Lester to the site several hours before we were scheduled to arrive, just to be sure that he did not miss an opportunity to meet a group of old men with diabetes wearing spandex who were tired but upbeat after riding bicycles across the country.

Lester was the only child in his school to have diabetes. Neither the school principal nor the staff were trained or prepared to handle this matter. His school did not have a full-time qualified nurse trained to care for a student with diabetes. Lester was very despondent and felt bad about himself. We did not know this when we were introduced to him. We greeted him as though we had known him forever. He watched as the entire squad took out their meters and tested in public—right there in the parking lot—and teased each other about our blood glucose readings. This got Lester smiling and laughing with us. Mom said that this was the happiest he had been since being diagnosed. We were not sure if meeting us uplifted Lester's spirits, or if it was the team baseball cap we gave him. At the end of the penalty timeout, we were off to complete the race. Meeting Lester was certainly one of the highlights of the race.

There were many other inspiring people. We met two four-man teams from Germany who were athletes without the use of their lower extremities due to paraplegia of the spinal cord. They used specially designed hand cycles to race across the country. They were led by their healthcare professional (also with paraplegia) who recruited and trained the team. He also led the fundraising activity to obtain the cycles and bring the team and crew to California. They were an inspiration to the other RAAM participants and spectators.

Then there was Dave. Dave was a sixty-nine-year-old racer who was a solo rider and, with the support of his crew, completed the race. Dave was not diagnosed with diabetes but had broken his back earlier in his career and needed modifications to his bicycle, which he designed in order to compete. This included a chin and back support mechanism that allowed him to climb the hills and mountains from a standing position. Dave endured plenty of pain and agony, but he was driven by his determination to complete the race. He succeeded in his mission.

My Special Team Member

Thinking back, I was fortunate to have had several outstanding team members on my side. This was not limited to RAAM and the other competitive events, but also included the healthcare professionals, friends, family, and all others who are struggling with our disease. However, there really is one special team member who made the greatest contribution. That is my wife, Eileen, who has shared my life for the past fifty years. If we include the time we met and dated from our high school years, we are talking about sixty years. We provided each other with the care and support to raise a family and to handle life's challenges as the years rolled on. Eileen had successfully figured out how to lose weight and maintain weight loss without yo-yo dieting. She made good food choices, watched our portion control, exercised, and followed a healthy life style. It has been a bonus for me to have Eileen in my corner. She loves life and intends to be around for a long, long time. Sort of the same thing I promised our grandson.

When I was diagnosed with diabetes, we both learned the best ways to prepare foods to control blood sugar, weight, and blood pressure. For Eileen, that was easy. She had already adopted those techniques and proved that they worked. In short, you can train yourself to eat the correct number of calories and carbohydrates to help control your blood sugars and to maintain your ideal weight. You can adopt a healthy lifestyle. Over time, not overnight, the body will seek its proper weight and maintain it for life. You are not really on a special diet; you are just eating the way we all should be eating to stay healthy.

The Benefits to Being a Person with Diabetes

Being diagnosed with diabetes is certainly not a death sentence. However, I thought it was right after my diagnosis. It took me some time to recognize that there are benefits and that it really was up to me to obtain them. Diabetes provided the motivation to live a healthier lifestyle in order to enjoy my family as they grew up and to actively participate in family matters. I now understand that the purpose of having and raising children is for them to give us grandchildren. I am getting ready to take my grandson on his first major group bicycle ride. Next year, I hope to take him on a multi-day bicycle tour. I look forward to doing the same with my granddaughter when she gets a little older. I hope to be able to fulfill my promise to my grandson and to my family that I will be around for a long, long time to come.

I have worked hard to do the right things to control my diabetes through lifestyle changes. I have been challenged to reach goals that I believed to be otherwise not obtainable. My most significant challenge was to learn portion control and to identify and avoid the "trigger foods" that threw me off track. My wife was the king pin for the nutrition and weight loss. I also increased my physical activity and discovered that I liked it to the point where I longed for the exercise sessions. I am not a skilled athlete; in fact, I am a bit clumsy, but I crave the rush of exercise-driven endorphins. I learned that it was all about activity and not the podium finish that produced the benefit. My physical activities grew to include running, resistance training and, of course, cycling. The benefits of exercise have been well documented, and I would like to add my "Amen!"

Having diabetes motivated me to lose weight (seventy-nine pounds over a three-year period) which helped me to keep the diabetes under control, lower my blood pressure and become a healthier me. As I see it, diabetes gave me the opportunity to join Team Type 2 and to participate in the Race Across America. Diabetes can be a difficult condition to manage and can be extremely frustrating if you try to do it by yourself. I certainly came from the school of "I can do this without help; I got into this myself and I will figure this out. Do I really need help?" Maybe! Consider your options. Do you really need to go this route on your own? Wouldn't it be helpful to share the burden and allow others to share your success? Why not consider building your own success team? Welcome those who can help you, make a contribution to your team, and be a contributor to another. Just recognize that you are the captain/CEO of your team!

Acknowledgment: I'd like to thank my wife Eileen, my daughter Karen, and Team Type 2 teammates for their support and editing of this chapter.

www.teamtype1.org